THE
PUBLIC
HEALTH
PRIMER

For Rick and Janislee
for their unending patience and support,
and for all the students who assisted along the way.

THE
PUBLIC
HEALTH
PRIMER

Jo Fairbanks
William H. Wiese

 SAGE Publications
International Educational and Professional Publisher
Thousand Oaks   London   New Delhi

For information:

SAGE Publications, Inc.
2455 Teller Road
Thousand Oaks, California 91320
E-mail: order@sagepub.com

SAGE Publications Ltd.
6 Bonhill Street
London EC2A 4PU
United Kingdom

SAGE Publications India Pvt. Ltd.
M-32 Market
Greater Kailash I
New Delhi 110 048 India

Printed in the United States of America

Library of Congress Cataloging-in-Publication Data

Fairbanks, Jo.
    The public health primer / by Jo Fairbanks and William H. Wiese.
        p.   cm.
    Includes bibliographical references and index.
    ISBN 0-7619-0652-5 (cloth).—ISBN 0-7619-0653-3 (pbk.)
    1. Public health.   I. Wiese, William.   II. Title.
    RA425.F25 1997
    362.1—dc21   97-21134

This book is printed on acid-free paper.

98 99 00 01 02 03 04 10 9 8 7 6 5 4 3 2 1

Acquiring Editor:	Daniel T. Ruth
Editorial Assistant:	Anna Howland
Production Editor:	Sherrise M. Purdum
Production Assistant:	Karen Wiley
Typesetter/Designer:	Yang-hee Syn Maresca
Cover Designer:	Candice Harman
Print Buyer:	Anna Chin

Contents

Preface

The *Public Health Primer* has been written to provide a basic introduction to public health. It makes the basics of public health accessible and understandable. It is a primer, and, as such, does not attempt an in-depth presentation of the basic concepts. Nor is it a general reference attempting to address all elements within the field. Instead, topics have been selected particularly to orient the reader to the field and demystify many of the concepts and technical terms that are commonly encountered in public health.

The Public Health Primer discusses both the science and application of public health. It is our hope that readers will come to understand that these are interdependent and each is essential to public health practice. Health planning and intervention rest on the science of epidemiology. The usefulness of epidemiology depends on what is done to improve health status after the statistics are compiled. Most important, readers need to understand that public health activities occur in a social and political environment that is constantly changing.

The Public Health Primer will be useful to anyone wishing to gain a quick overview of the basics of public health. The book is appropriate for undergraduate students in the health sciences, health education, nursing, pharmacy, and allied health. It may be appropriate for graduate students pursuing advanced degrees in these areas as well as in medicine, health administration, health policy, public administration, and public health itself. It will be helpful for the many workers employed within the public health sector who have never had an opportunity to gain perspective on the overarching principles basic to this field.

Jo Fairbanks, Ph.D.
William H. Wiese, M.D., M.P.H.

Part I

THE HISTORY, DEVELOPMENT, AND ORGANIZATION OF PUBLIC HEALTH

Activities currently carried out under the label of public health are varied and complex. People employed in public health practice can be found working in the areas of epidemiology, statistics, monitoring and surveillance, infectious and chronic disease control, health education, health promotion, violence and tobacco and substance abuse prevention, maternal and child health, adolescent health programs, environmental protection, mental health, aging, and international assistance, among others. Public health workers are employed in federal, state, and local governmental agencies as well as in private and not-for-profit organizations. What is meant by public health, and how did public health activities become so seemingly diverse? Why are there so many different agencies and organizations engaged in improving the public's health?

This section briefly reviews the history and development of public health practice. It examines how the focus of public health has changed over the years as the factors that influence health and illness have changed. This evolution has, as its foundation, action taken to protect and enhance the health of the population. Public health occurs in a social context. Its responsibilities have evolved throughout history to meet the demands of people in societies who take steps to reduce threats to health and to become healthier through organized individual and community action. The study of the history of public health also demonstrates that public health practice is not static and will certainly continue to change.

This section examines the concepts of health and public health, the evolution of health protection activities, and the current organization of public health in the United States. It also presents a framework for understanding public health activities, which organizes those efforts under the three core functions of assessment, policy development, and assurance.

Chapter 1

History and Development

⎯⎯⎯⎯⎯⎯⎯⎯⎯⎯ ⚬⚬ ⎯⎯⎯⎯⎯⎯⎯⎯⎯⎯

Definition of Health and Public Health

Any discussion of public health must be preceded by definitions of *health*. Just what constitutes health has long been debated. Over the years, in fact, the definitions of health have changed. The word health is derived from the old English word "hal" meaning hale, whole, healed, sound in wind and limb (Last, 1987, p. 5).

Past definitions have included idealized views of health such as that of the *World Health Organization (WHO)*: "A state of complete physical, mental, and social well-being, not merely the absence of disease or infirmity" (WHO, 1944, p. 29). This view of health as an ideal condition is also found in standard dictionary definitions, which refer to health as the "condition of being sound in body, mind, or spirit; freedom from physical disease or pain" (*Merriam Webster's Collegiate Dictionary*, 1990, p. 558).

More recently, however, viewing health as an ideal, ultimate state or perfect condition has evolved into a view of health as a continuum that recognizes that perfect health may be unattainable. Health is now recognized to be a dynamic state that changes depending on the degree of adverse factors affecting the individual. Viewing health as a dynamic process adds a degree of flexibility so that individuals can see themselves at different stages of health at different times.

In 1986, the WHO developed a new definition of health that recognizes the interaction between individuals and their environments: "The ability to identify and to realize aspirations, to satisfy needs, and to change or cope with the environment. Health is therefore a resource for everyday life, not the objective of living. Health is a positive concept emphasizing social and personal resources, as well as physical capabilities" (WHO, 1986, p. 426). Within this definition, health can be understood to be part of an ecological relationship, an interrelatedness between the individual and the environment. It is now widely recognized that the health of an individual depends on biology, personal health habits, and a competent medical system, and also on a safe environment and supportive living conditions that enable individuals to realize aspirations.

Public health, like health, is also slowly evolving toward a "process" definition. Traditional definitions emphasized the role of government in protecting the public's health, a social action.

C. E. A. Winslow (1920) defined public health in 1920 in terms of targeted activities: "the science and art of (a) preventing disease, (b) prolonging life, (c) and organized community efforts for sanitation of the environment, control of communicable infections, education of the individual in personal hygiene, organization of medical and nursing services for the early diagnosis and preventive treatment of disease, and the development of the social machinery to ensure everyone a standard of living adequate for the maintenance of health, so organizing these benefits as to enable every citizen to realize his birthright of health and longevity."

"Public health is one of the efforts organized by society to protect, promote, and restore the people's health. It is the combination of sciences, skills, and beliefs that is directed to the maintenance and improvement of the health of all the people through collective or social actions. . . . Public health activities change with changing technology and social values, but the goals remain the same: to reduce the amount of disease, premature death, and disease-produced discomfort and disability in the population. Public health is, thus, a social institution, a discipline, and a practice" (Milbank Memorial Fund Commission as cited in Last, 1995, p. 134).

The goal of public health is to protect the community against the hazards engendered by group life. Public health is "public" because its activities are community centered involving organized community effort (Institute of Medicine, 1988, p. 39).

The Future of Public Health was issued in 1988 by the Institute of Medicine (IOM), a private, nonprofit organization that provides health policy advice under congressional charter to the National Academy of Sciences. This report proposes a three-part definition for public health. The mission of public health is the fulfillment of society's interest in assuring the conditions in which people can be healthy. The substance of public health is organized community efforts aimed at the prevention of disease and promotion of health. It links many disciplines and rests on the scientific core of epidemiology. The organizational framework of public health encompasses both activities undertaken within the formal structure of government and the associated efforts of private and voluntary organizations and individuals (Institute of Medicine, 1988, pp. 40-42).

The role of government in public health varies. In many countries health resources development, services delivery, and financing are under the control of a national governmental agency. Socialized governments such as China and Cuba maintain almost exclusive, central control over health care delivery. Others, such as the British national health service and Norway's Ministry of Social Affairs, have strong roles in planning and managing health care delivery but also have organized systems for regional and local input. In the United States, there is no single federal agency that oversees the health care system. The writers of the U.S. Constitution, perhaps more concerned with the guarantee of individual freedoms than providing for the social welfare, did not mention health. A strong, market-driven, private medical care system, financed largely by individuals, not government, has flourished. In the United States, governmental public health activities have largely developed independently of a centralized plan from one exclusive agency, but, rather, have responded to more local needs to protect and improve the public's health.

History of Public Health: Emergence of Disease Control

Today's public health activities have roots in ancient history. That history evolved from early attempts to protect the members of the tribe, the society, and the community. Even without a thorough understanding of the causes of illness, early humans, led by empirical evidence, took certain measures to protect the public's health. Survival, for example, would have been clearly enhanced by uncontaminated water and food, and prohibitions against "fouling" the environment would have resulted in healthier people. Over time, the importance of sanitation would emerge as the central goal in the control of infectious disease.

Evidence of sanitation efforts has been found in very early civilizations. An ancient city built over 4,000 years ago in the north of India at Mojenjo-Daro had paved streets covering sewers that drained bathrooms located in well-built houses (Rosen, 1993).

The Minoan and the Mycenaean cultures, both ancient Aegean civilizations (3000-1500 B.C.) had public water systems, drainage canals, and flushing toilets. Palaces, such as Knossus on the island of Crete, had ornate bathing facilities promoting cleanliness, which was highly regarded for health protection.

The influence of the subsequent 2,000 years of the classic Greco-Roman civilization cannot be overemphasized. During this period, many of the world's great religions came into being, and the foundation was laid for art, science, mathematics, medicine, and astronomy. Greek thinkers looked for logical explanations for what they observed. This thinking changed perceptions about the causes of illness. Sickness was no longer viewed as being caused by demonic possession but, rather, as a natural sequence of conditions that could be explained. Natural treatment for illness was widely practiced (Palmer & Colton, 1995).

The growing cities of the Greek and Roman civilizations were supplied with fresh water via aqueducts for use in bath houses, fountains, and public buildings. Roman engineering skills provided cities with roads and with sewage systems that are still in use today. The Roman aptitude for government, law, and administration made management of the cities in a widespread empire possible (Palmer & Colton, 1995). Officials were appointed to protect the public's health by providing for garbage collection and disposal, street cleaning and repair, and cleaning of the public bath houses and latrines. A system of inspection ensured oversight of public taverns and inns as well as building construction and removal, thus beginning current public health activities in food and environmental protection (Rosen, 1993).

The Middle Ages, or medieval period (500-1500 A.D.) was characterized by the further growth of cities. Commerce flourished, although aggression was also common, and cities fortified their boundaries to provide for the public's defense. Sanitation and maintenance of a pure, ongoing supply of water and food provided challenges to people who lived with their animals inside walled fortifications (Rosen, 1993). Efforts in public health expanded in the Middle Ages as city administrators struggled to reduce the increasing pollution of a burgeoning population. Poor and often undernourished people were crowded together in unsanitary conditions, which assisted the rapid spread of disease.

During the medieval period, leprosy spread from Egypt to Europe. Cholera, smallpox, measles, and bubonic plague swept across continents every few years killing thousands with each wave. Ongoing epidemics of infectious disease resulting in high rates of mortality were commonplace in Asia and Europe (McNeill, 1989).

By the 1300s, plague spread westward until it reached the Black Sea, and then traveled by ship and caravan to all the parts of the known world with a devastating impact. By 1340, 13 million people in China had died, and India was almost depopulated. Pope Clement VI reported that half of the world's population of approximately 43 million people had died, and the plague returned again and again. In 1348, Europe lost millions as the Black Death attacked Paris, London, Venice, and Florence (Hecker, 1839). Entire towns were lost and cultivated fields were abandoned for lack of workers. Famine killed many who had survived the disease (see Figure 1.1).

Leprosy, as well as the plague, was epidemic in communities in the Middle Ages. Much earlier, the Hebrews, as recorded in Leviticus, had recognized that lepers had a transmissible disease that could be passed to healthy persons and consequently ordered their isolation. Medieval communities reacted in similar ways. Lepers were considered a public menace and banned from the community forever. Leprosaria, or leper houses, were placed far outside the boundaries of the communities and lepers were forced to wear a special costume and warn others of their presence (Rosen, 1993, pp. 40-41).

When the plague repeatedly spread throughout the world during the Middle Ages, city officials used the knowledge they had gained from the isolation of lepers to protect the populace from this new dreaded disease. Plague victims were isolated and their houses quarantined.

Because ships increased the possibility of contact with the plague bacteria through infected sailors, rodents, and fleas, public health measures such as quarantine laws for seaports became commonplace. The word *quarantine* means a 40-day period, which was the standard length of time that seaports began to restrict incoming ships and travelers from entry. Places of isolation for the sick, later known as hospitals, were developed in the Middle Ages. The effectiveness of these measures was often enhanced by the unintended consequences of changes in living conditions. For example, in Europe, as stone houses with tile roofs replaced wooden, thatched-roof dwellings, the black rat, a common carrier of the plague bacteria, had less access to the population (McNeill, 1989).

In addition to expanded activities in disease control, public health administration also grew during the Middle Ages. Public health activities continued to focus on the supply of clean water, refuse disposal, the cleanliness of the city and the marketplace, and the quality of the food supply, but these activities became more formally organized.

Millions of Persons

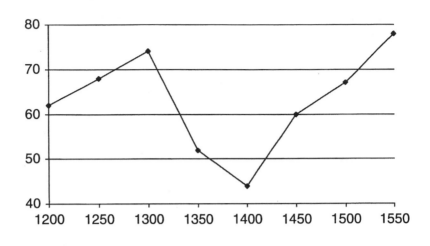

Figure 1.1. The Approximate Population of the World, 1200-1550 A.D.
SOURCE: Bennett (1954).

Formal organization was necessary, in part, because of the then widespread belief that disease resulted from the decay of organic matter or from stagnant water, which caused the air to become virulent. This corrupt air, when breathed in, attacked the humors of the body. Corrupt air was associated with decaying food, increasing the city's responsibilities for protecting the consumer in the medieval marketplace, the most important public gathering place. Because spoiled food was seen as harmful, great care was taken to prohibit the sale of objectionable meat and fish. Markets were cleaned each evening and refuse disposed of. In medieval Zurich, for example, fishmongers were required to get rid of dead fish that had not sold during the day (Rosen, 1993, pp. 34-35).

The modern public health practices of food inspection, the regulation of its sale, and the licensing and monitoring of food sellers can be traced from the Roman Empire through the medieval marketplace to cities today. Current ongoing public health activities to assure the purity of drinking water, adequate refuse disposal, and disease preven-

tion all have their roots in ancient history. Many of these accomplish-
ments took place without a thorough understanding of the nature of
disease, and, as knowledge of disease developed, public health practice
continued to evolve.

The Rise of Microbiology in Disease Control

With the Renaissance (1450-1600) came the beginnings of science.
Copernicus, Galileo, and Leonardo da Vinci changed the thinking of
the Middle Ages. Art, literature, and architecture were nurtured, and
trade and commerce flourished. The population of Europe began to
increase and a renewed curiosity about the causes of disease opened a
new era of exploration. By the middle of the 16th century, leprosy,
plague, tuberculosis, scabies, smallpox, influenza, and syphilis had
been identified as separate diseases with their own distinct symptoms.

The Atlantic Ocean, previously a barrier, became a starting point
for navigation that circled the globe. The colonization of America by
Europeans resulted in armed conflict and conquered peoples. Human
violence proved to be not as destructive as epidemic disease, which
resulted in depopulation for natives with no resistance to European
diseases (Palmer & Colton, 1995). In 1518, smallpox reached His-
paniola and only 1,000 natives survived, according to Bartoleme de
Las Casas. From there it spread to Mexico, where it devastated the
Aztecs, and later to Peru, where it rendered the Incas vulnerable to
subjugation (McNeill, 1989, pp. 183-185).

In the early 1600s, Athanasius Kircher (1602-1680) and Antony
van Leeuwenhoek (1632-1723) used microscopes to initiate a new
method of scientific study. Leeuwenhoek succeeded in seeing bacteria,
protozoa, and red blood cells, but did not suspect their role in disease.
Kircher claimed the plague was caused by minute living organisms.
His work attracted followers looking for disease germs, but it was not
until the 1800s that the germ theory was revived (Rosen, 1993).

Early attempts to protect against smallpox in Europe included the
direct inoculation of matter from a pustule into a small lesion on the
recipient's skin. Some developed severe cases of the disease through

this method and died, but most had light cases and were, thus, protected from contracting the disease in its more virulent form. Edward Jenner (1749-1823), a physician in Britain, successfully vaccinated a boy against smallpox using cowpox matter. Cowpox was not a serious disease in humans, and the new method of vaccination became common and acceptable. These advances contributed to public health prevention activities, but progress beyond those of basic quarantine was slow (McNeill, 1989). Only in the 20th century, with the emergence of immunobiology as a science, would immunization yield large-scale public health benefits.

Industrialization and Social Change

As medical technology advanced so, too, did the theories of mercantilism and economic development. The welfare of society seemed to be improved with increased wealth and power, and nations moved toward trade and industrialization. A large and healthy population was needed to supply the workforce, and activities in compiling census and health statistics were undertaken. John Graunt was a pioneer in developing quantitative measures of death in populations. His classic book, *Natural and Political Observations . . . on the Bills of Mortality*, appeared in England in 1662. In it, he noted the deaths due to physical, mental disorders, and accidents; the ratio of births to deaths; the excess of urban over rural death rates; and the differences in the seasonal death rate (Rosen, 1993, p. 88). Following Graunt's work and others, record keeping on the population began in earnest as an interest in the health of the population reemerged as a highly valued condition. Today's health monitoring and surveillance activities that assess the health of the public are based on these early beginnings.

Unfortunately, conditions in the cities of Europe were such that maintaining an adequate standard of living was a challenge to the masses of people living there. As industrialization spread, more people moved to the cities for work, and the crowded and difficult living conditions led to ongoing epidemics and high morbidity rates and mortality rates among the working class. Even today, urbanization in economically emerging nations continues on a massive scale along with similar attendant problems.

By the 19th century, throughout Europe, serious efforts at the reform of the existing social conditions were begun. In 1842, public health reformer Edwin Chadwick's famous *Report on an Inquiry Into the Sanitary Conditions of the Laboring Population of Great Britain* was published. Chadwick pointed out that more than half of the children of the working classes died before their fifth birthday, and that in the industrialized cities of England the average life span for the gentry was 36 years, 22 years for tradesmen, and 16 years for laborers. As a consequence of this report, a General Board of Health for England was established followed by the appointment of the first medical officer for health for London. As the roots of reform took hold and London struggled to provide pure water and adequate sewage disposal, legislation was passed on child welfare, management of pollution, and care of the aged and infirm. London became an example for other European cities, often leading the way in public health and social reforms (Richardson, 1887).

In colonial America, Boston, New York, Philadelphia, and Baltimore had established boards for health by the late 1700s. Their primary responsibility was to provide disease protection, pure water supplies, and sanitation. Port cities were exceptionally challenged to provide health protection for citizens due to the constant arrival of travelers. Merchant seamen were frequently injured or ill, while also poorly paid and without a permanent home. Port cities did not relish taking responsibility for poor, ill seamen, and their complaints resulted in the U.S. Congress passing the Marine Hospital Service Act in 1798. The Act required a tax of 20 cents per month per seaman to be paid to the tax collectors in the port cities, which, in return, provided for "the temporary relief and maintenance of sick or disabled seamen in the hospitals or other proper institutions" (Williams, 1951).

The tax to support the Marine Hospital Service Act was placed in the Treasury Department of the federal government, and as the demand for services increased, the department provided financing for increasing numbers of physicians and later hospitals to meet the need. This growing demand for services resulted in what eventually became a cadre of physicians and several public hospitals in the Marine Hospital Service, later known as the U.S. Public Health Service.

By the 1800s, the growing responsibilities under the direction of public health now included the provision of medical care to those who could not access the existing health care system. Personal health care services were provided first to merchant marines and later other special populations such as the urban poor, poor mothers and children, American Indians, and others. The next chapter describes how these beginnings evolved into the current systems of public health in the United States.

Chapter 2

The Current
U.S. Public Health System

In the United States during the 19th century, the responsibilities of the Marine Hospital Service continued to increase. The medical director of the service, originally appointed in 1870, became known as the *surgeon general*. The newly named Public Health and Marine Hospital Service was organized formally under his direction. By 1912, the service was reorganized and renamed the United States Public Health Service. It was not until the 1930s that the Public Health Service was moved from the Treasury Department into a new Federal Security Agency by President Franklin D. Roosevelt. Later, the Federal Security Agency became successively reorganized as the Department of Health, Education, and Welfare and later as the *Department of Health and Human Services (DHHS)*. The Public Health Service (PHS) is currently located organizationally under the DHHS.

In the United States, unlike many other countries, there is no constitutionally mandated system for public health. Rather, public health activities have grown to meet the demands of a society when it finds threats to its health unacceptable. As threats to health evolve, the management of some of these threats is best accomplished at the local level, whereas others are best controlled at the state or national level. During the 1900s, the role of public health agencies greatly expanded. Although the federal government undertook more responsibility for the public's health and safety, local and state departments of health were also growing.

In general, over the years, the role of health departments at all levels moved beyond the control of food, water, sanitation, and disease into gathering and compiling health statistics, health planning, financing and pro- vision of health services, and regulation and licensing of service providers and facilities. Overall, the investigation of the cause and spread of disease and the dissemination of health information still forms the core of public health activities, but today's national, state, and local health departments provide a large variety of functions. Table 2.1 illustrates the mission and essential services of public health.

Federal Health Agencies

Federal departments and agencies with health-related activities and roles include the Department of Health and Human Services, which houses the *Health Care Financing Administration (HCFA)*—responsible for administering *Medicare* and *Medicaid* and certifying clinical laboratories, and the *Public Health Service* (PHS); the Department of Agriculture; the Department of Labor; the regulatory authority for workplace health and safety; the Department of Defense, which provides health care for the armed services; and the Environmental Protection Agency (EPA).

There are often multiple agencies operating within the same general area of concern. For example, assurance of the purity and safety of the nation's food supply can involve federal, state, and local public health agencies—each performing a distinct and vital service. The U.S. Department of Agriculture (USDA) inspects and grades meat through its Food Safety and Inspection Bureau. Other USDA bureaus monitor

TABLE 2.1　Public Health Mission and Services

Mission
Promote Physical and Mental Health and Prevent Disease, Injury, and Disability

Public health
- Prevents epidemics and the spread of disease
- Protects against environmental hazards
- Prevents injuries
- Promotes and encourages health behaviors
- Responds to disasters and assists communities in recovery
- Assures the quality and accessibility of health services

Essential public health services
- Monitor health status to identify community health problems
- Diagnose and investigate health problems and health hazards in the community
- Inform, educate, and empower people about health issues
- Mobilize community partnerships to identify and solve health problems
- Develop policies and plans that support individual and community health efforts
- Enforce laws and regulations that protect health and ensure safety
- Link people to needed personal health services and assure the provision of health care when otherwise unavailable
- Assure a competent public health and personal health care workforce
- Evaluate effectiveness, accessibility, and quality of personal and population-based health services
- Research for new insights and innovative solutions to health problems

NOTE: • = Adopted by the Public Health Functions Steering Committee (1994). Committee members included the American Public Health Association, Association of Schools of Public Health, Association of State and Territorial Health Officials, Environmental Council of the States, National Association of County and City Health Officials, National Association of State Alcohol and Drug Abuse Directors, National Association of State Mental Health Program Directors, Public Health Foundation, U.S. Public Health Service (Office of the Assistant Secretary for Health, Agency for Health Care Policy and Research, Centers for Disease Control and Prevention, Food and Drug Administration, Health Resources and Services Administration, Indian Health Service, National Institutes of Health, and Substance Abuse and Mental Health Services Administration).

and control animal and plant diseases to protect the health of consumers. Additives to any food product are controlled by the U.S. *Food and Drug Administration (FDA)*, an agency of the Public Health

Service, which requires proof that food additives do not harm consumers. State departments of health oversee food safety through licensure and inspection of public facilities. Local health departments monitor the safety of the food supply through inspection of food service facilities. Local health inspectors assure that establishments that serve, prepare, and distribute food are periodically examined for cleanliness and safety of food handling and preparation. Thus, a broad range of agencies make it possible to be reasonably confident that the food purchased, prepared, and served by a local restaurant is indeed safe for consumption.

Even though a myriad of federal agencies are involved in health to some degree, the primary responsibility for public health at the national level rests with the Department of Health and Human Services (DHHS). The head of the DHHS is a cabinet-level secretary who is appointed by the president. Within the DHHS, the Public Health Service includes the Office of Public Health and Science and the following operating divisions: (a) the *Centers for Disease Control and Prevention (CDC)*, (b) the *Food and Drug Administration (FDA)*, (c) the *Health Resources and Services Administration (HRSA)*, (d) the *National Institutes of Health (NIH)*, (e) the Substance Abuse and Mental Health Services Administration, (f) the Agency for Toxic Substances and Disease Registry, (g) the Agency for Health Care Policy and Research, and (h) the *Indian Health Service (IHS)* (see Figure 2.1).

The mission of the CDC is to promote health and quality of life by preventing and controlling disease, injury, and disability. The CDC monitors health by assessing and compiling health statistics on the U.S. population. It is the epidemiology unit for the nation. The CDC collects, analyzes, and disseminates health information. It oversees a national system for disease surveillance and conducts research and laboratory screening. It is actively involved in environmental health, occupational health and safety, disease prevention, health promotion and education, and technical assistance to state and local health departments and other countries. The CDC plays a vital role in the nation's public health activities.

The NIH, the largest PHS agency, is the principal biomedical research arm of the public health service, conducting its own research

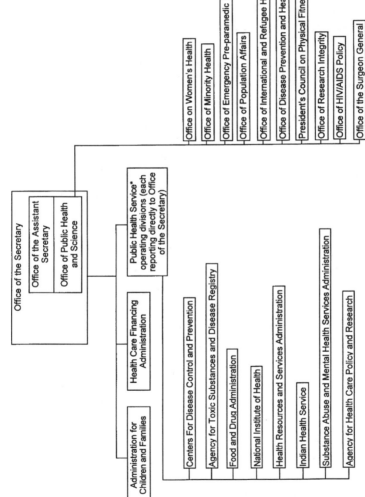

Figure 2.1. Department of Health and Human Services and Offices of the Public Health Service

NOTE: The Public Health Service is comprised of the Office of Public Health and Science and its 10 offices, the 8 operating divisions, and the Regional Health Administrators (not shown).

and providing grant support for others' research. NIH includes 17 separate health institutes, for example, the National Cancer Institute, as well as the National Library of Medicine and the National Center for Human Genome Research. NIH employs more than 16,000 workers and provides billions of dollars for biomedical research projects.

The FDA regulates the use of drugs, food substances, and other consumer goods, requiring proof that products are safe for the consumer. The FDA requires clinical testing to approve substances but does no testing on its own. For drugs or food additives to enter the marketplace, a complex approval process, which can take years and cost millions of dollars, must be followed.

The Health Resources and Services Administration (HRSA) funds a broad variety of programs that support the health professions and the delivery of service, especially to underserved areas and populations. Health care delivery services are not supplied directly through the agency, but are supported indirectly through the *National Health Service Corps*, for example, among others.

Grants-in-Aid

Although some federal agencies, such as the Department of Veterans Affairs—which oversees a large system of medical services for veterans and is a separate department that is not part of the DHHS—and the Indian Health Service, do supply clinical services, most federal activities in health care take place through grants and contracts to others. Federal grants-in-aid are the primary vehicle for the national government's role in health care. Grants-in-aid promote revenue sharing among the federal, state, and local governments while achieving federal government goals and objectives through grant requirements. Over the years, Congress has continued to supply funding through block and categorical grants to special populations and areas of concern. *Block grants* are those funds generally organized into broad categories such as maternal/child health, substance abuse and mental health, preventive health, and primary care. The state governments receiving block grant dollars have a great deal of control over expenditures of those dollars as long as basic federal requirements are met. A *categorical grant,* on the other hand, can be more restrictive in nature, allowing little local control. For example, a categorical grant might fund a specific project for measles immunization that would have very detailed requirements for project implementation and evaluation.

One very important factor influencing the growing diversity of public health activities has been the grants-in-aid funding projects. As more state and local public health institutions reached out for federal dollars, public health activities moved steadily toward an emphasis on those special populations and categorical concerns. Today, most health departments will have ongoing programs in maternal and child health including nutrition and immunization, tuberculosis, sexually transmitted disease, dental health, mental health, and substance abuse among others—all major concerns funded over the years through grants-in-aid. The extent to which a somewhat unifying public health policy in the United States exists is primarily through the use of federal grants-in-aid to the states to achieve national goals.

State and Local Departments of Health and Other Public Health Providers

The states are principally responsible for the health of the public residing within their boundaries. Each state has a slightly different method of approaching public health concerns, but most states engage in activities similar to those illustrated in Table 2.1. Whether through block grants, categorical grants, or legislative funding, state departments of health carry out national and state mandates; manage environmental, educational, and personal health services; collect, analyze, and disseminate health information; respond to statewide health crises; set public health policies and standards; inspect; and conduct health planning and evaluation (Institute of Medicine, 1988, p. 173).

Total expenditure for government public health activities in 1995 was $31.4 billion (see Chapter 3), of which all state and local agencies spent $27.6 billion (Health Care Financing Administration, 1997). Most of the total public health expenditure is for individual health care services. In 1997, the Public Health Service (PHS) and the Public Health Foundation reported the results of an eight-state survey to determine the states' expenditures for the essential public health services (see Table 2.1). Of the total funds spent by the states on all public health activities, personal health care services accounted for 69% of the total. Of the expenditures for personal health care services, 70% were spent for mental health. The findings indicate a predominance of personal health care services in the public health systems of the states, with more than $2 of every $3 expended in this category. Spending for community-based services accounted for only 1.2% of the total (Centers for Disease Control and Prevention [CDC], 1997a).

There are basically two organizational models for state health departments. One is that of a separate agency that reports directly to the governor. The other is as a component of a larger "superagency," such as a Department of Health and Environment or Health and Human Services. Most states have reorganized over the years so that their Departments of Health are independent and freestanding. Most are directed by a secretary or commissioner of health who is assisted by chief medical officers, most of whom have medical degrees. Of the states, 24 have boards of health that oversee health financing and policy development (Institute of Medicine, 1988, p. 173).

Local health departments are responsible for the delivery of services mandated by statute, which usually include control of communicable disease, environmental protection, health education, and management of health data and information. They can be independent or part of the state departments of health. There are regional, county, and city health departments, and they differ in size, organization, jurisdictions, programs, and populations served. Directors of local health departments are chosen by the unit of government they serve. Mayors, city managers, city and county boards and councils, and state department directors can appoint local health office directors. Approximately one third of states have local "field" offices that are an extension of the state department. Another one third are responsible to local government and the state health department, and one third are autonomous, responsible only to local government or the local health board (Institute of Medicine, 1988).

There are also private and professional, nongovernmental organizations involved in public health. Examples are the American Heart Association, the American Cancer Society, Alcoholics Anonymous, Association of Retarded Citizens, American Public Health Association, and many others organized around certain diseases or concerns.

Foundations, such as W. K. Kellogg, Robert Wood Johnson, Pew Trust, and Kaiser Family Foundation, provide millions of dollars to support health research and community health activities that improve public health. These private foundations are an important part of public health activities, and are instrumental in shaping health policy in the United States (Institute of Medicine, 1988, p. 194).

"The public's health depends on the interaction of many factors; thus, the health of a community is a shared responsibility of many entities, organizations, and interests in the community, including health service delivery organizations, public health agencies, other public and private entities, and the people of a community" (Institute of Medicine, 1996, p. 1).

Chapter 3

Public Health Practice: Assessment, Policy Development, and Assurance

***

Over the years, as reported in Chapter 2, a major role for public health agencies has become that of direct service provider. It has been argued that public health agencies should be engaged in the prevention of disease and not so much in its treatment. Yet, providing care for the nation's 40 million uninsured has not been addressed since efforts at health care reform failed in 1994. This has become an increasing problem for public health policymakers. Who should provide access to quality health care for the uninsured? In this era of cost containment, can market forces be expected to solve the current dilemma of financing personal care for the growing numbers of uninsured? What is the future role for public health?

National health care expenditures have been rising somewhat alarmingly over the past two decades. Total spending in 1995 was $988.5 billion (see Figure 3.1). This amount represents 13.6% of the

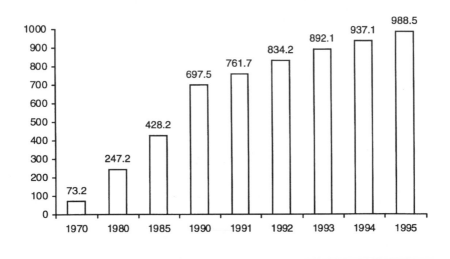

Figure 3.1. National Health Expenditures, 1970-1995 (in billions of dollars)
SOURCE: Health Care Financing Administration (1997).

U.S. gross domestic product (GDP) (see Figure 3.2), considerably more than any other developed country spends for health care. As illustrated in Figure 3.3, spending for health care services and supplies was dominated by hospital care and physician services, which consumed 55% of the total. Government spending for health care, primarily for Medicare and Medicaid, has increased each year, reaching 46.2% of total expenditures in 1995, as seen in Figure 3.4 (Health Care Financing Administration, 1997).

Concern over health care spending is centered on the large portion of the GDP it takes. This affects both private and public financing systems. Resources are not unlimited and governments, as well as corporations, must decide how to apportion available funds. In government, when health care costs take ever larger percentages of the budget, less money is available for other programs, such as education or defense. Private companies are affected by rising health care expenditures when the cost of providing coverage for workers rises. Profits, and the ability to increase salaries, are reduced. The necessity of passing on these costs to the consumer can affect economic competitiveness.

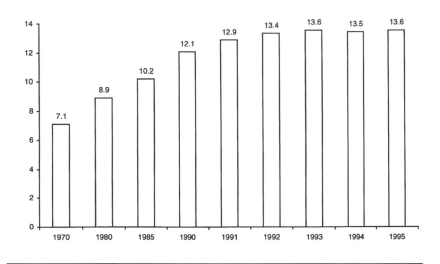

Figure 3.2. National Health Expenditures, 1970-1995, Percentage of Gross Domestic Product
SOURCE: Health Care Financing Administration (1997).

Efforts to reduce the costs of health care have resulted in several strategies undertaken by both government and private organizations. A fixed, diagnosis-related hospital payment system was initiated by Medicare in 1983 as a cost control measure to curtail "fee-for-service" reimbursement. Fee-for-service financing had reimbursed providers for the total cost of the patient's care, with few limitations on the medical interventions. The Medicare Prospective Payment System (PPS) established a rate of payment based on specific patient problems and standard or average costs incurred in the treatment of the problem. These diagnosis-related groups, or DRGs, categorized and established flat payment rates for more than 400 medical conditions. Hospitals treating Medicaid and Medicare patients, for example, were no longer automatically reimbursed for the full cost of patient service but, rather, for the prospectively determined amount only. This provided an incentive to reduce hospital length of stay and costs. Payment based on DRGs continues to be a widely used cost control method.

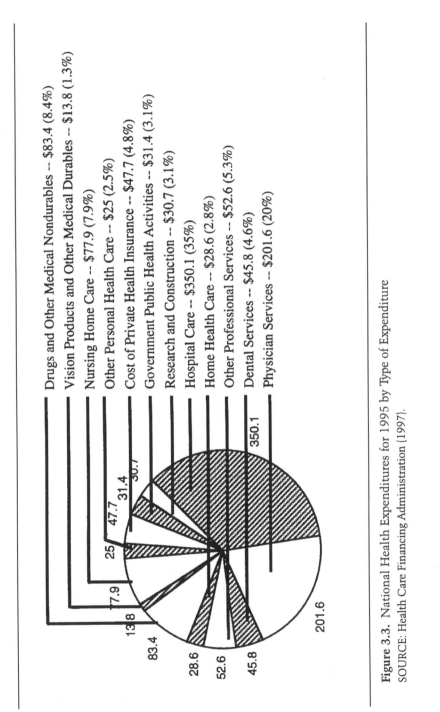

Drugs and Other Medical Nondurables -- $83.4 (8.4%)

Vision Products and Other Medical Durables -- $13.8 (1.3%)

Nursing Home Care -- $77.9 (7.9%)

Other Personal Health Care -- $25 (2.5%)

Cost of Private Health Insurance -- $47.7 (4.8%)

Government Public Health Activities -- $31.4 (3.1%)

Research and Construction -- $30.7 (3.1%)

Hospital Care -- $350.1 (35%)

Home Health Care -- $28.6 (2.8%)

Other Professional Services -- $52.6 (5.3%)

Dental Services -- $45.8 (4.6%)

Physician Services -- $201.6 (20%)

Figure 3.3. National Health Expenditures for 1995 by Type of Expenditure
SOURCE: Health Care Financing Administration (1997).

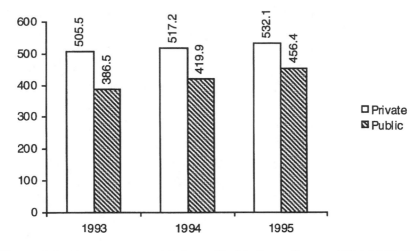

Figure 3.4. Government and Private Health Expenditures, 1993-1995 (in billions of dollars)
SOURCE: Health Care Financing Administration (1997).

Capitation is a certain fixed per-patient amount negotiated with a health care system by corporations or insurance companies, for example, to provide care for individual patients for a period of time such as one year. Capitation is rapidly becoming the most common form of health care payment to hospitals and large health care delivery systems. Under capitation, the *risk* of losing money, resulting from a population that incurs costs beyond what was predicted, can be passed from the insurance company to the provider (Tabbush & Swanson, 1996).

Managed care organizations (*MCO*) are under the management of a single entity that insures members, furnishes benefits through a defined network of providers, and manages the practice of those providers (Institute of Medicine [IOM], 1996, p. 13). Managed care systems such as *health maintenance organizations* (*HMO*) and preferred provider organizations (PPO) use primary care physicians as "gatekeepers" to control the patient's access to specialty services and medical tests and procedures (Tabbush & Swanson, 1996). The management places limits on providers and patients alike. Patients are restricted to a certain network of providers and hospitals, and providers are restricted in their use of diagnostic tests or specialty treatments.

As the health care delivery system changes, there are few data on quality and satisfaction with managed care. The data that do exist indicate that hospitals, in a competitive situation, are unwilling to pass on the costs of treating the poor, called cost shifting, to insured patients. Market-driven health care may make the system more efficient, but it does not make it easier to provide care for the poor and uninsured (Preston, 1996).

As organized health care delivery systems increase and provide care for a growing number of people, it may be possible for public health agencies to partner with the private sector in new ways. Clearly a more coherent and comprehensive system of providing personal health care services for the uninsured is needed. Redefining the role of public health may be necessary. What are the core functions of public health that should remain the responsibility of government public health agencies?

To answer this question, the Institute of Medicine (IOM) convened the Committee for the Study of the Future of Public Health in 1986. The committee assignment was to assess the status of governmental public health practice at that time, and make recommendations that would guide future policy and public health practice. Its report, *The Future of Public Health* (IOM, 1988), has had an enormous impact on the structure and substance of governmental public health in the United States. Recently, the IOM established the Committee on Public Health to review the progress that has been made in the decade since the report was issued. The Committee on Public Health's analysis indicates that "the concepts in *The Future of Public Health* remain vital and essential to current and future efforts to energize and focus the efforts of public health. These concepts need to be advanced, applied, and taught to all health professionals" (IOM, 1996, p. 5).

In the original report, the Committee for the Study of the Future of Public Health saw the government role in public health as being made up of three functions: assessment, policy development, and assurance. Because of its importance, this chapter draws directly from that report.

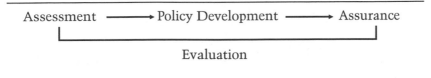

Figure 3.5. The Government Role in Health Assessment Policy Development Assessment Evaluation

Assessment

This heading includes all the activities involved in the concept of community diagnosis—such as surveillance, identifying needs, analyzing the causes of problems, collecting and interpreting data, case finding, monitoring and forecasting trends, research, and evaluation of outcomes.

Assessment is inherently a public function because policy formulation, to be legitimate, is expected to take in all relevant available information and to be based on objective factors, to the extent possible. Private sector entities are expected to have self-interests. Therefore the information they generate, although frequently quite useful to the policy process, is not judged by its fairness. In contrast, although public agencies in practice do not always weigh all sides of a question, in principle they are obligated to do so.

Moreover, public decisions take place in the context of limited resources. Society cannot do everything it would like to do or with the intensity it might prefer. Thus trade-offs among competing uses of resources are necessary. The wisdom, justice, and perceived legitimacy of public decisions are crucially affected by the quality of the information on which they are based. A function of government is to provide a central mechanism by means of which competing proposals can be assessed equitably. . . .

The assessment function facilitates good decisions in both the private and public sectors. Because assessment seldom has its own constituency, however, it is often starved for resources. A fully developed assessment function is an absolutely essential part of the ideal public health system, and it is one that the committee believes to be in large measure attainable.

Policy Development

Policy formulation takes place as the result of interactions among a wide range of public and private organizations and individuals. It is the process by which society makes decisions about problems, chooses goals and the proper means to reach them, handles conflicting views about what should be done, and allocates resources. Government provides overall guidance in this process. In contrast to private entities, it alone has the power to give binding answers. Therefore, although it joins with the private sector to arrive at decisions, government has a special obligation to ensure that the public interest is served by whatever measures are adopted. As with other governmental entities, the public health agency bears this responsibility. . . . It must raise crucial questions that no one else raises . . . and strive for fairness and balance.

The public health agency should be equipped for this role by its technical knowledge and professional expertise. Used judiciously, the knowledge base of public health tempers the excesses of partisan politics and makes for more just decisions. Technical knowledge will have the best effect, however, when used in the context of a positive appreciation for the democratic political process, by professionals who are politically as well as technically astute.

Assurance

The assurance function in public health involves seeing to the implementation of legislative mandates as well as maintaining statutory responsibilities. It includes developing adequate responses to crises and supporting crucial services that have worked well for so long that they are now taken for granted. It includes regulating services and products provided in both the private and public sectors, as well as maintaining accountability to the people by setting objectives and reporting on progress. Assurance implies the maintenance of a level of service needed to attain an intended impact or outcome that is achievable given the resources and techniques available.

Carrying out the assurance function requires the exercise of authority. This is not a responsibility that can be delegated to the private sector. Members of society expect government to make certain that they enjoy at least adequate safety and security. The public health agency must be able to exercise authority consistent with fulfilling citizens' expectations and must account to them for its actions with equal energy.

As part of the assurance function, in the interest of justice, public health agencies should guarantee certain health services. Such a guarantee expresses a measurable public commitment to each member of society. In operational terms, this implies guaranteeing both that the services are available (present somewhere in the community) and, in the case of services to individuals, that the costs will be borne by the government for those unable to afford them. When these services are not and cannot be present in the larger community, it is the public health agency's responsibility to provide them directly. . . .

In recent years a competitive market approach to the provision of health services has been advanced as the potential solution to ills that plague the U.S. health system, cost inflation in particular. While recognizing the existence of competition in service delivery, the committee believes that the responsibilities outlined must be exercised by government to ensure basic capacity throughout the system. (Reprinted with permission from *The Future of Public Health*, © 1988 by the National Academy of Sciences. Courtesy of the National Academy Press, Washington, D.C.)

Further recommendations from the Committee on Public Health, 1996, conclude that public health agencies and organized health care systems must reach agreement on roles and responsibilities; governmental public health agencies should increase their ability to oversee health care providers and become equal partners with insurance regulators and Medicaid agencies; public health professionals should be further educated and trained to work with health services organizations to ensure quality personal health services in communities; public health should work with all entities that influence health in a community toward enhancing health; and, that environmental regulation and enforcement of public health laws must remain the responsibility of governmental public health agencies (IOM, 1996, p. 3)

Part II

BASIC CONCEPTS AND ANALYTICAL TOOLS IN PUBLIC HEALTH

Public health seeks to promote health and control disease. To do this successfully, it is necessary to understand what actually determines health status and what underlies, or causes, disease. This is true whether one is addressing infectious disease, chronic disease, or mental health. The determinants are almost always multifactorial. There are biological and behavioral determinants, and environmental and social determinants may underlie either of these. Chapter 4 presents a model of disease that facilitates understanding of the role of determinants and introduces the science that seeks to understand determinants—epidemiology. Additional discussion of determinants as applicable to global health issues is given in Part III, Chapter 11.

The assessment functions in public health involve the analysis of data gathered through surveillance, the identification of need, examination of the factors contributing to health problems, research, and other means that shed light on the health problem. Objective interpretation of accurate data is necessary before appropriate intervention can take place. Without the tools of assessment, monitoring, and interpretation, rational public health practice would not exist.

Chapters 5 and 6 examine the assessment tools of public health. These chapters introduce some of the terms and methodological approaches commonly used in descriptive and analytical epidemiology. These approaches are used to build the scientific basis necessary to understand the determinants of health and disease. Chapter 7 describes ways in which these are applied in public health practice.

Chapter 4

Epidemiology and the Determinants of Disease

Approaches to preventing disease or controlling its spread depend on identifying the determinants and understanding how they may most effectively be addressed. A *determinant* of disease is anything that is causally associated with the disease. The science that permits understanding and rational decision making in public health is *epidemiology*. Epidemiology is the systematic, objective study of the natural history and distribution of health-related conditions in populations, and the factors that determine their occurrence and spread (Terris, 1985).

Model of Disease

A disease occurs in a person (*host,* or victim). The disease may have an immediate *cause* that is readily understood. Tuberculosis is caused by a bacterium, *Mycobacterium tuberculosis*. Malaria is caused by a parasite that infects blood cells and damages organs in the body. Some injuries are caused by a moving object striking the victim. The moving object may be a falling rock, an automobile, or a bullet. In these examples, the bacterium, the parasite, and the moving objects are *agents*. Agents reach hosts in a variety of ways. In malaria, the parasite is transmitted from person to person by mosquitoes. The mosquito is a *vector*. A vector is that which carries or transmits the agent to the host. Tuberculosis is transmitted directly from one infected and contagious person to another person.

These elements—host, agent, and the environment in which they interact—constitute the beginning of an explanatory model depicting how disease occurs (MacMahon & Trichopoulos, 1996, chap. 2). The model originated in describing infectious diseases. It can apply to the description of chronic diseases as well. With cancer, for example, the affected host is the person with cancer. The agent might be a chemical *carcinogen* or ionizing radiation. Cigarettes can be viewed as a vector in transmitting carcinogens found in tobacco smoke. For many chronic diseases, there is no one essential agent; rather, the disease emerges when multiple causal factors interact with the host, often in a complex manner.

The host and agent interact in time and place and within an environment (see Figure 4.1). The causal factors, or determinants, may be viewed as residing with the host, the agent, or the environment or, as is often the case, with some combination. There are many aspects to environment: geographic, physical, chemical, and biological, to name just a few. The environment may affect the host-agent interaction in many ways and provide opportunities for intervention to prevent or slow the spread of disease. The transmission of malaria provides an example. The climate and geographic environment affect whether or not the species of mosquito that carries malaria can breed. An intervention to prevent malaria might be to eliminate standing pools of water, which are needed for breeding. Another approach could be to use mosquito netting to provide a barrier that keeps the mosquito away from the host.

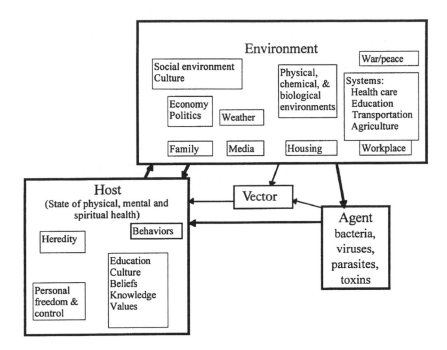

Figure 4.1. Examples of Relationships Among Host, Agent, and Environment

There are other types of environment that can be important in health and illness, such as occupational environments that might include the presence of work site chemicals and dangerous equipment. Social environments can also increase the likelihood of exposure to infectious or other toxic agents through crowded housing and the absence of safe water and food.

A determinant may be a necessary and sufficient element, such as the bacterium *M. tuberculosis*, without which no one would get tuberculosis, or it may be only contributory. Contributory factors for tuberculosis include those that affect the susceptibility of the host, such as nutritional status and immune status. Other contributory factors include environmental situations that influence exposure of the susceptible host and transmission of the bacterium, such as crowding and poor air circulation.

Host-related determinants influence susceptibility, and include genetic or immunologic conditions and behaviors such as using tobacco, alcohol, and drugs, and participating in sexual behaviors that lead to infection or unwanted pregnancy.

Environment can influence host risk behaviors. The social environments of advertising and peer pressure influence the likelihood that a child will adopt smoking or alcohol use. Stress, absence of social support, and unemployment are *risk factors* for many diseases. Socioeconomic class influences the likelihood of disease and death independently of other known risk factors. Thus, the economic and social environments are also extremely relevant to health.

As chronic disease and violence have gained ascendancy as major causes of mortality, refinements in the model of disease stress the interaction among factors. In the web of causation model, disease is viewed as developing through interconnecting chains of causation in which each element is the result of a complexity of antecedents (MacMahon & Trichopoulos, 1996, chap. 2).

The role of the epidemiologist is to study all the factors that might be determinants. Identification of determinants is essential to the development of rational strategies for prevention and control of disease. Considerable amounts of public health resources have been directed at conducting epidemiologic studies. (Chapter 6 describes some of the approaches epidemiologists use in identifying the determinants and making causal inferences.) It is important that the full range of determinants be studied. It is not enough to identify just the immediate cause. As noted, the bacterium *M. tuberculosis* is a necessary and sufficient cause of tuberculosis. Understanding this as the cause, however, does not alone result in control of this infection. The availability of excellent antibiotics for the treatment of tuberculosis is insufficient to control the spread of the disease. Other factors critically affect the management of the disease and must be viewed as contributing causes. Contributing determinants of tuberculosis include the difficulty in engaging many persons with active disease in effective treatment programs; loss to follow-up of patients needing prolonged treatment; the interaction of HIV infection with the activation and spread of tuberculosis; and persistence of poverty, malnutrition, and inadequate housing in many population groups.

The systems of determinants range hierarchically from the global to the proximate. The metaphor of the Chinese boxes, or a set of nested boxes, has been suggested as a way to understand the complex relationships of disease to determinants and of the determinants to each other. "The outer box might be the overarching physical environment, which, in turn, contains societies and populations (the epidemiological terrain), single individuals, and individual physiological systems, tissues and cells, and finally (in biology) molecules" (Susser & Susser, 1996, p. 676).

Examples

The following examples of diseases and conditions illustrate how identification of the determinants helps point the way for prevention or control. Each is an important cause of mortality. One is an infectious disease (*HIV/AIDS*). Two are chronic diseases that have behavioral and social determinants (lung cancer and coronary heart disease). Tobacco use is also included separately. Itself a behavior, it has its own determinants and is viewed by Centers for Disease Control and Prevention (CDC) as a notifiable condition. Homicide is not a disease in the customary sense of the term, but represents a cause of death that is potentially preventable.

HIV/AIDS. AIDS is the eighth leading cause of death in the United States and leading cause of death for those aged 25-44 years (CDC, 1996a). There is abundant evidence that AIDS is caused by the human immunodeficiency virus (HIV). The emergence of the AIDS epidemic in the 1980s presumably followed the adaptation of this virus from animal hosts to strain(s) pathogenic to humans. Although HIV is necessary for contracting the disease, there are many contributing factors. The public health challenge has been to identify the determinants that promote the transmission of the virus. The virus is transmitted through sexual contact, direct injection by way of contaminated needles and transfusion of contaminated blood products, and from mother to fetus or newborn at birth. Because some of these routes derive from personal behaviors, preventive strategies have emphasized education about avoiding or modifying behaviors to reduce the risks of transmission, such as condom usage and use of sterile needles. Identification and treatment of pregnant women having HIV infection offer the opportunity to reduce rates of infection of the baby. There are also social determinants that influence the risk behaviors in ways that promote disease transmission and undermine efforts at preventive education. For example, high rates of HIV infection in Africa are thought to derive from aspects of the culture and economy. These include the frequent use of prostitutes by men, resistance to use of condoms, and the dominance by the male with respect to sexuality within marriage. The political environment, including the hesitation of some governments to publicly acknowledge the spread of HIV in their countries and initiate aggressive preventive action, has often permitted the disease to spread unchecked. Societal prejudice against some of the population groups at greatest risk has contributed to governmental failure to assign to AIDS the kind of public health priority afforded to other threats from infectious disease.

Lung cancer. Cancer of the lung has a poor prognosis even when diagnosed at seemingly early stages. Studies on the effectiveness of screening people for detection and treatment of early lung cancer have failed to demonstrate reductions in subsequent death rates. Routine screenings using chest x-ray or sputum cytology are not presently recommended (U.S. Preventive Services Task Force, 1996). Lung cancer is noteworthy, however, in that there are very effective ways of reducing the likelihood of its occurrence. By far the most significant determinant for lung cancer risk is smoking tobacco. Environmental exposures also associated with lung cancer include exposure to carcinogens in environmental tobacco smoke, radon gas, various other chemical carcinogens, and asbestos. Identification of these agents along with understanding how they work and how exposures occur provide the bases for preventive intervention.

Biological differences between people influence who will develop cancer at any given level of exposure. Theoretically, preventive interventions might be constructed to reduce the host's biological susceptibility, for example, through genetic engineering or through other chemical enhancements. At present, such individually targeted, biologically based interventions remain either undeveloped or unproved. Most currently adopted strategies depend on the separation of people from carcinogenic agents. For the individual, this means addressing behaviors such as tobacco use and avoidance of situations where exposure to carcinogens may occur. At a social level, strategies seek to reduce the presence of the carcinogenic agent or the circumstances where people can be exposed, such as efforts to reduce the promotion and availability of tobacco and to regulate chemical hazards in the workplace.

Coronary heart disease (CHD). Although CHD has afflicted humans for a very long time, its occurrence ballooned in the 20th century, making it the number one cause of death in most developed and some developing countries. Some people have a hereditary predisposition for CHD, and it affects males at an earlier age than females. Females develop a pattern of increased risk after menopause. Replacement of estrogen after menopause appears to be protective against CHD. Individual susceptibility is also tied to biologically measurable risks, including abnormalities of blood lipids, hypertension, distribution patterns of body fat, and increased blood homocysteine and ferritin. High rates of CHD can be tied to behavioral determinants. Most important among these are the use of tobacco and eating and exercise behaviors. Diets with large amounts of certain kinds of fats and sedentary behaviors promote risk conditions such as obesity, the expressions of adverse lipid profiles, high blood pressure, and diabetes. Each of these conditions can contribute to the development of CHD and to the abnormalities of clotting associated with the eventual clinical manifestation of this disease in susceptible persons. Stress may have a role in the pathogenesis of the CHD as well as in the timing of its clinical manifestations. Lack of social support and lower socio-economic status are also associated with CHD independently of other factors listed. The culture, economy, and public policies that enable and promote personal risk behaviors must themselves be considered as determinants of the CHD epidemic.

The reduction of CHD mortality (49% between 1972 and 1992 in the United States, as reported by the *National Center for Health Statistics*) reflects the combined effects of decreased incidence and, among those with disease, improved survival. The decline in incidence rates has been associated with reduction of risks in the population, particularly tobacco use in adults, control of high blood pressure, and reduced consumption of certain dietary fats. Also contributing to reduced mortality have been improvements in the emergency services and the clinical management of life threatening events associated with CHD, such as heart attack and long-term treatments to reduce recurrence (Hunink et al., 1997).

Public health strategies for intervention range from dealing directly with individuals with respect to risk behaviors and risk conditions; dealing at a community level with the social environments that promote these behaviors; and public policies that influence, for example, the availability, promotion, and use of tobacco and foods that contribute to harmful levels of blood lipids.

Tobacco use. Over 400,000 deaths annually in the United States are attributable to tobacco use (U.S. Department of Health and Human Services, 1989). Smoking is, of course, a behavior and not a disease in the usual sense. Because of its enormous importance, the Centers for Disease Control and Prevention (CDC) has begun listing it among the disease conditions it routinely monitors and tracks (CDC, 1996b). Cancers, *cardiovascular disease (CVD)*, and lung disease are only three of the numerous serious types of diseases that can result from tobacco use. Substances in tobacco smoke work in the body at the cellular level to produce immediate physiologic effects, which can result in damage to lungs and vasculature or in cancerous changes. Exposure to nicotine results in biological dependency and biological reinforcement of smoking behavior. Although there is individual variation in susceptibility to the harmful effects of the biologically active and carcinogenic substances in tobacco smoke, there is no effective means to reduce individual susceptibility or mitigate the effects from exposure.

Smoking is a behavior. Individuals choose to initiate this behavior and, to the extent that choice is possible in the face of addiction, choose to maintain the behavior. The choice to smoke is heavily influenced by environmental determinants. These include the media and social and cultural influences. These in turn are affected by promotional efforts of tobacco producers and actions or inaction of governments and regulatory agencies. The prevalence of smoking varies with socioeconomic status, and efforts to combat tobacco use that are targeted only at behavior change will be limited in their effectiveness.

> Any meaningful public health intervention regarding tobacco must also consider why manual workers smoke more than nonmanual workers and find it more difficult to give smoking up and why most physicians have responded to the epidemiologic evidence and given up smoking, whereas nurses continue to smoke in great numbers. . . . When a public health problem is studied in individual terms (e.g., tobacco smoking) rather than in population terms (e.g., tobacco production, advertising, and distribution, and the social and economic influences on consumption), then it is very likely that the solution will also be defined in individual terms and the resulting public health action will merely move the problem rather than solve it. (Pearce, 1996, p. 680)

Homicide in youths. Because it involves actions, violence with intentional physical injury (homicide, assault, rape, and domestic violence) is not a disease in the usual sense. It is handled through the criminal justice system rather than the health care delivery system. Violence, however, may be considered as a health condition, may be interpreted within the frame of the model of disease, and studied with epidemiologic tools.

Homicide rates in the United States rose rapidly during 1979-1992 (see Figure 4.2), especially in urban areas, and enormously exceed corresponding rates found in other countries (see Figure 4.3). A decline in rates occurred in 1995, but homicide remains the 12th leading cause of death overall in the United States, and the leading cause of death among African Americans aged 15-24 years (CDC, 1996a).

Approaching intentional injury using a disease model has proven to be beneficial. The host must be viewed as both the perpetrator and as the victim. The agent is the means of injury, for example, a handgun or other weapon. The environment is the physical, domestic, or greater social context that influences the violent act.

Youths at risk for committing homicide are more likely than others in the population to be male, young, and a minority (African American, Hispanic, Native American); have a history of prior crimi-

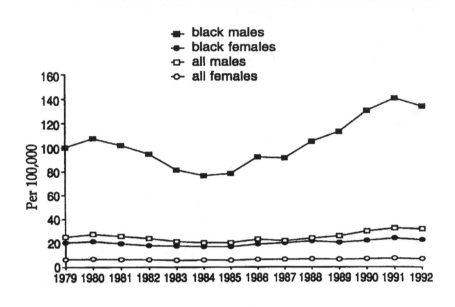

Figure 4.2. Homicide Death Rates for Americans, 15-34 Years, 1979-1992
SOURCE: Centers for Disease Control and Prevention/National Center for Health
Statistics, National Vital Statistics System, 1979-1992.

nal behavior, have been a victim of violence; and live in poor, urban
settings. Homicide is likely to occur when alcohol or drugs have been
used. Lack of impulse control is considered to be a factor. Another
factor is the availability of firearms, which enhance the lethality of
violent behavior and account for 7 out of every 10 murders.

Sorting through the numerous and tangled variables of youth
homicide is a daunting task. The epidemiology needed to fully understand its determinants is far from complete. The excess proportion of
minorities involved probably reflects the racial composition of poor
urban neighborhoods. The extent to which handguns are carried may
reflect in part an attempt at a protective response to living in a
threatening environment, rather than simply being the contributor to
the initiation of the violence. Proposed intervention strategies include
restrictions on the access to and the carrying of firearms; teaching
skills in nonviolent conflict resolution; control of domestic violence

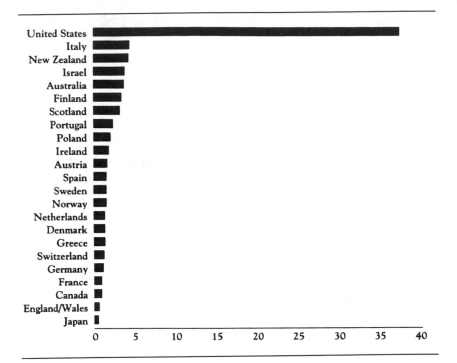

Figure 4.3. International Variation in Homicide Rates for Males, 15-24 Years, 1988-1991
SOURCE: Mercy, Rosenberg, Powell, Broome, and Roper (1993); data from the National Center for Health Statistics; World Health Organization.

and its perpetuation onto others by its victims; and steps to alleviate the crowding, poverty, alienation, and helplessness associated with life in the urban ghetto.

Determinants and Causes of Death

In public health, identifying the causes of death is useful to the extent that it helps lead to preventive action. In this respect, classifying causes of death in terms of the disease or conditions that result in death, as tabulated from death certificates (see Chapter 7), is important, but only as a first step. The diseases that cause the most deaths

**TABLE 4.1   The Ten Leading Causes of Death as a Percentage of
All Deaths: United States, 1900 and 1993.**

1900	Percentage	1993	Percentage
Pneumonia	11.7	Heart diseases	33.1
Tuberculosis	11.3	Cancer	23.9
Diarrhea and enteritis	8.3	Stroke	6.5
Heart diseases	8.0	Bronchitis and emphysema	4.2
Stroke	6.2	Injuries	4.0
Liver disease	5.1	Pneumonia and influenza	3.5
Injuries	4.2	Diabetes	2.3
Cancer	3.7	HIV infection	1.6
Senility	2.9	Suicide	1.4

SOURCE: Centers for Disease Control and Prevention (1995a, p. 7).

**TABLE 4.2   Leading Causes of Death Expressed as Risk Factors
and Agents in the United States in 1990**

	Deaths	
Risk Factors and Agents	Estimated Number	Percentage
Tobacco use	400,000	19
Diet/activity patterns	300,000	14
Alcohol use	100,000	5
Microbial agents	90,000	4
Toxic agents	60,000	3
Firearm use	35,000	2
Sexual behavior	30,000	1
Motor vehicles	25,000	1
Illicit use of drugs	20,000	<1

SOURCE: McGinnis and Foege (1993).

change over time. In the United States, the most common causes in
1900 and in 1993 are shown in Table 4.1.

Some fraction of the individual diseases that lead to death may be
attributable to specific risk factors. Another way of analyzing the
causes of death, then, is to look at the risk factors that account for the
diseases and conditions that lead to the deaths. (The concept of
attributable risk is discussed in Chapter 5 and the concept of assigning
causation is discussed in Chapter 6.) Expressing causes in terms of

risk factors has the advantage of making explicit what might be targeted in an intervention. Table 4.2 shows one attempt to look at the causes of death in the United States in this manner and purports to account for half of all deaths in terms of addressable risk behaviors or environmental circumstances.

Additional Reading

Lilienfeld, D. E., & Stolley, P. D. (1994). *Foundations of epidemiology* (3rd ed.). New York: Oxford. (See chapter 3.)

Chapter 5

Basic Measurements and Statistics

————————— ✿ —————————

To track a disease or any sort of health problem in a population requires that observations be organized and expressed in language that is meaningful to others. Terms that are commonly used by epidemiologists and public health workers are introduced in this chapter. Many of these terms are used in later chapters of this book. These terms need to be understood to respond critically to information about public health issues. Also addressed is the use of *statistics* in the interpretation of quantitatively expressed information and inferences. This chapter offers an introduction to technical materials. Readers who wish to explore the subject in greater depth should consult one of the texts listed under Additional Reading.

Case Definition

A person identified as having a disease is referred to as a *case*. To deal with any measurement of diseases or to study determinants, one needs to be able to identify the cases with some acceptable degree of reproducible accuracy. This is not always easy to put into practice. Many symptoms and signs associated with a disease are nonspecific, occurring in association with any number of different diseases or conditions. Commonly encountered examples of nonspecific signs of illness are fever and cough. Fever can occur in association with a large number of different infections. Cough can be from respiratory infections due to a variety of agents, from noninfectious irritants, or from medical conditions such as chronic pulmonary disease and cancers. Other examples of nonspecific signs include weight loss, vomiting, and abdominal pain. If one is trying to study the determinants of a disease, it is important that the identified "cases" are true cases of the disease. In practice, the epidemiologist works with the clinician to establish an operational *case definition*. To the extent that the definition is specific, the epidemiologist is helped in identifying critical determinants, such as a specific infectious agent. To the extent that other diseases are included among the true cases, the epidemiologist's ability to assess specific determinants will be weakened. In this context, the epidemiologist may want a case definition that is as precise as possible. Once a disease has been characterized and investigators have developed diagnostic tests that are specific and sensitive, the positive diagnostic test itself may become an important component of the case definition.

Consider the example of HIV/AIDS. When what we now understand to be AIDS first became apparent, epidemiologists were working only with what was an excessive incidence of Kaposi's sarcoma (a distinctly unusual form of cancer that is evident on the skin), serious infections due to organisms that typically would not occur except in persons who have poor immunological defenses, or both. Initially, most victims were identified as homosexual males. The initial case definition became being homosexual and having at least one of these conditions. By careful study of persons fitting this profile, investigators determined that this acquired immunodeficiency syndrome (AIDS) was a transmissible condition that affects the immune system, including loss of the normal concentration of T4 cells in the blood. The same cluster of symptoms (*syndrome*) was discovered in drug users who shared needles and in some persons who had received transfusions of blood. Depression of T4 cell count was added as an element within the case definition. Using rigorous case definitions, scientists were able to link AIDS with infection with a previously unknown virus, which they named human immunodeficiency virus (HIV). With techniques to identify persons infected with HIV, investigators could screen persons for HIV and study the natural history of the infection and its more subtle manifestations.

As another example, in a community in New Mexico, people became concerned with what appeared to be an excess incidence of brain cancers, thinking that these might be tied to an environmental hazard. On careful investigation, some of the "cases" proved not to have been primary brain cancer or even proven cases of cancer at all. By deducting these false cases, the apparent excess was substantially reduced. The residual excess has been studied, but no common exposure has been identified. The excess may simply have been a chance occurrence. The initial anxiety about a possible outbreak of cancer was accentuated by the lack of a specific case definition.

Screening and Testing for Disease

In identifying persons with disease, some sort of testing is usually required. Tests may be either screening or diagnostic. Screening tests generally are relatively crude tests that attempt to identify persons who are likely to actually have the disease. Confirming the presence of the disease requires additional testing with diagnostically specific tests. A concern about the use of either a screening or a diagnostic test is the ability of the test to accurately identify the condition.

Sensitivity. Sensitivity is a measure of the capability of finding all cases of a designated condition. The term is used in the context of both screening and diagnostic tests. A test with a sensitivity of 100% would detect all cases. A test with a sensitivity of 75% would identify three fourths of the cases.

TABLE 5.1   Relationship Between Sensitivity and Specificity

	Disease Present	*Disease Not Present*
Test positive	**a** True positive	**b** False positive
Test negative	**c** False negative	**d** True negative
	a + c All cases	**b + d** All noncases

Sensitivity:	Proportion of all cases detected as positive by test: a / (a + c)
Specificity:	Proportion of all noncases detected as negative by test: **d / (b + d)**
Predictive value of a positive test:	Proportion of all positive tests that are true positives **a / (a + b)**
Predictive value of a negative test:	Proportion of all negative tests that are true negatives **d / (c + d)**

$$\text{Sensitivity} \quad = \quad \frac{\text{Number of true cases identified}}{\text{Total number of cases}}$$

Specificity. Specificity is a measure of the capability of a test to exclude (fail to identify as positive) noncases. If a test has a specificity of 100%, all cases found will be true positives. To the extent that a test is nonspecific, some of the instances of identified cases will in fact not be true cases. These are called *false positives.* (This does not mean, however, that all true positives will be identified. That would happen only if this test were also 100% sensitive.) If a test has specificity of 90%, then 90% of all noncases would be correctly identified as negatives. This means, however, that 10% of the negatives will be misidentified as positive (false positives). The relationship between sensitivity and specificity is summarized in Table 5.1.

In the context of screening for a condition that is infrequent in the population being screened, lack of high specificity in the test will result in a large proportion of the persons with positive tests being false positives. In such situations, a positive test is said to have a low *predictive value* in terms of indicating a true positive case.

It would be unusual for a test to have perfect sensitivity or perfect specificity. Consequently, there will almost always be some proportions of tests that are false negative and false positive.

Frequently, as a test is refined or adjusted to be more sensitive, it loses specificity. Conversely, as a test is made to be more specific, it will become less sensitive. Choices depend on the needs of the situation, as is evident in the following three situations pertaining to screening for HIV/AIDS. At a blood bank, it is imperative that as many HIV positive donors as possible be excluded from donation to avoid the catastrophe of transmission of the deadly infection by way of contaminated blood products. Accordingly, prospective donors and the blood donated are screened with the most sensitive tests available. Such screening maneuvers may be relatively nonspecific so that there will be true HIV negative donors excluded among the positives. The situation is different for testing to diagnose HIV infection for clinical purposes. Persons actually infected with HIV should be correctly identified (sensitivity) to be able to offer counseling and timely treatment. Also, however, it could be personally disastrous to misidentify and mislabel a person as having HIV infection when that is in fact not the case. Thus, clinical testing for HIV must be highly specific as well as sensitive. This is achieved by applying a sequenced, double test in which the initial screening component is sensitive but inadequately specific. Blood samples that are positive at this initial stage are then confirmed with more highly specific testing. A third situation might be in a research setting where investigators seek to characterize some aspect of persons infected with HIV, for example, response to a new treatment. Here the priority will be on having a highly specific case definition, and sensitivity will be of secondary importance.

Measures of Occurrence

Data illuminating health problems must be presented so that others can understand their importance. Counts of the numbers of cases are not meaningful without a standard of comparison. For that reason, simple, numerical counts are expanded into rates that include a consideration of the population as well as a time frame for the event. The rates have as their denominator a standard of comparison that makes sense.

Incidence. Incidence is the rate of occurrence of new cases of a specified condition in a specified population within some specified period of time (most often a year):

$$\frac{\text{Number of new cases occurring}}{\text{Average number of persons in population}}$$

Incidence is usually arithmetically converted to express the rate as being per 1,000, 10,000, or 100,000 population. This permits direct comparisons of rates across different populations.

Prevalence. Prevalence is the proportion of a specified population with a specified condition at a given point in time:

$$\frac{\text{Number of persons with the condition}}{\text{Number of persons in the population}}$$

As with incidence, prevalence is arithmetically computed to be expressed as the number per 1,000, 10,000, and so on. For any given incidence rate, a disease that is chronic, slowly fatal, or both will have a greater prevalence than one that is self-limited or rapidly fatal. This is because cases of the former will accumulate in the population.

Mortality. Mortality rates are measures of the incidence of death. Overall mortality is the incidence of death in the entire population. *Infant mortality* is the incidence of death in babies aged from birth to one year. *Case fatality* is the proportion of cases that die from the disease.

Crude and Adjusted Rates

The direct measure of a rate, such as incidence, in a population gives a value that is called a *crude rate.* Crude rates may be used to make a comparison across different populations or within a given population

over time, but only if the populations in question have similar characteristics. The following example illustrates what needs to be done
when the populations are dissimilar.

A comparison has been made of mortality rates from cancer in two
counties. Overall mortality is found to be twofold greater in County A
than in County B. It is not immediately certain, however, that the
people in County A are at excess risk. Suppose County A has a large
proportion of aged retirees. County B lacks a substantial retiree
population, having instead a large proportion of younger people.
Because older people are much more likely to get cancer and die from
it than are younger people, it is not surprising that the mortality
rate from cancer in County A is higher than in County B. To make a
meaningful comparison of the rates in the two counties, one has to
compute an *adjusted rate*. Age-adjustment is a process of comput-
ing observed rates separately for each age group within each county
and then using these rates to compute what would be the overall rate
in a hypothetical population having a standardized age profile. If sex
is a confounding determinant, one might compute age-sex-adjusted
rates. It would be only after adjusting for such differences in Counties A and B that one could derive a meaningful comparison between
the two. Comparison of crude, or unadjusted, rates can be quite
misleading.

Crude rates do serve as a direct measure of disease or death in the
community. This can be a useful measure if one is concerned with
allocating resources for the disease management. In the above example, one might allocate resources for management of cancer in
County A, even though individuals may not be at higher risk within
any age group.

Risk and Comparing Risks

Risk is the probability that something will occur in an individual over
the course of some period of time. Time needs to be specified. It may
be a year, 10 years, or a lifetime. It may also be some appropriate
postexposure period, such as the risk of an unimmunized person
getting measles after exposure to an active case. A risk of 100% (or

1.0) indicates that the outcome is inevitable. Risk is determined by observational studies in populations in which the incidences under various situations are noted. The risk to a given individual may be inferred from such observations. In applying information about risk to an individual, one has to be sure that the individual and his or her situation are similar to the circumstances present in the studied population.

Risk factors. A risk factor is something that, when present or applicable, is associated with increased risk for a disease. It may be increased genetic susceptibility, a risky behavior, or a particular environmental exposure.

Relative risk. Relative risk is the multiplier by which baseline risk is changed as a result of a specified determinant. The relative risk is determined directly by dividing incidence in a group exposed to a determinant by the incidence in a group that is without exposure to the determinant:

$$\frac{\text{Incidence in exposed population}}{\text{Incidence in unexposed population}}$$

It is important that the two comparison groups are otherwise comparable. To the extent that there are multiple other determinants that could confound the measure of relative risk, there are statistical techniques for adjusting for these, such as multivariate analysis.

A relative risk of 1.0 means that an exposure results in no change in incidence with respect to the baseline incidence rate, or a person is no more likely to get the disease. A relative risk greater than 1.0 indicates increased risk. A relative risk of 2.0 means the risk is doubled; a relative risk of 3.0 means the risk is tripled; and so on. A relative risk of 0.5 means the risk is halved; a relative risk of 0.25 means the risk is quartered; and so on. The relative risk for heart disease in the United States from smoking lies between 2.0 and 4.0, depending on the amount and duration of the smoking.

Attributable risk. Attributable risk is that part of the total incidence of a condition in an exposed population that is due (i.e., attributable)

TABLE 5.2 Death Rates[a] and Relative Risks of Death[b] From Lung Cancer in Males With Heavy Occupational Exposure to Asbestos and in Males Without Occupational Exposure, Tabulated by Tobacco Use

| | Occupational Exposure to Asbestos | |
Tobacco Use	None	Positive History of Exposure
Never a regular user	11.3 (1.0)	122.6 (10.8)
Regular user	58.4 (5.2)	601.6 (53.2)

SOURCE: Data from Selikoff and Hammond (1979).
a. Deaths are age-adjusted and expressed per 100,000 man-years of follow-up.
b. Relative risks of death appear in parentheses.

to exposure to a specific determinant: It is computed in exposed populations by subtracting what would have been the incidence if there were no exposure (determined from observations of unexposed populations) from the observed incidence in the exposed population:

$$\text{Attributional risk} = (\text{Incidence in exposed population}) - (\text{Incidence in unexposed population})$$

Consider the data shown in Table 5.2, regarding workers who have been occupationally exposed to asbestos. Attributable risks of the exposure to asbestos are calculated by doing the subtraction shown above. Among the nonsmokers, the attributable risk of lung cancer from occupational exposure to asbestos is 111.3 deaths per 100,000 man-years of follow-up. Among the smokers, the attributable risk is 543.2 deaths per 100,000 man-years. Relative to nonsmokers without occupational exposure to asbestos, the attributable risk of smoking and having exposure to asbestos is 590.3 deaths per 100,000 man-years. It is apparent from Table 5.2 that tobacco use and occupational exposure to asbestos are each associated with increased relative risk for lung cancer. When the two occur together, the risks are multiplied, not simply added—indicating a synergistic interaction between the two risk factors.

Attributable risk is a useful measure in public health because it conveys a sense of the achievable benefit in the exposed group if the exposure to a given determinant could be eliminated.

Population attributable risk. Attributable risk, described in the preceding subsection, is a computation of the added risk taken on among persons who have been exposed to a risk. Attributable risk does not take into account the prevalence of exposure in the greater population. The attributable risk for lung cancer from heavy occupational exposure to asbestos may be judged as being very high. If, however, there is little such exposure actually occurring in the general population, the overall risk from asbestos may be quite low. This is reflected by calculating the population attributable risk (PAR). PAR is computed by multiplying the attributable risk by the prevalence in the population of the those who are exposed, and dividing by the overall incidence.

$$\frac{(\text{prevalence of exposed persons}) \times (\text{attributable risk})}{(\text{overall incidence in the population})}$$

PAR is computed either as the fraction or as the percentage of total incidence that is attributed to the exposure. PAR is high when the prevalence in the population of those with the exposure is high, and when relative risk from the exposure is high. It is low when the prevalence is low. PAR is an extremely useful measure in public health planning, for it predicts the reduction in incidence that may be achieved if the exposure to the determinant or risk factor is reduced. Knowing the PARs associated with exposures to various risk factors can guide allocation of resources available for intervention.

Statistics

Statistics refers to the analytic tools that are essential for the applications of epidemiology and in the interpretation of data. Properly applied, statistical analysis gives the epidemiologist extremely valuable tools. Statistical tools are used to organize and analyze quantitative measures. With statistical analysis, researchers and epidemiologists are able to interpret the significance of differences observed across separate sets of measurements, express the strength of association between measures that correlate with each other, sort through complex sets of data, and dissect out how each of several variables might contribute to an observed outcome. Problems arise when the methods of statistics are improperly applied, the limits of statistical conclusions are overlooked, or the gathered data are in error or otherwise flawed.

Some aspects of statistics are familiar, such as the computation of an average to express a measure of central tendency within a group of measurements. Much of statistics, however, is quite technical, with concepts and methods that comprise a full course of study. The following introduces just a few concepts that commonly appear in general readings.

Statistical significance. Statistical methods allow us to understand the extent to which measured differences in two incidence rates may be consistent with being due purely to chance. Assessing the role of chance is done through statistical significance. A measured difference may be *statistically significant* if the likelihood of its being due to chance is very low. It will not be statistically significant if the difference could be due to chance rather than to real differences. Statistical methods permit computation of such probabilities. The statistical equations take into account the magnitude of the observed difference, the sizes of the samples used in determining the rates, and other factors. The measure of probability that a difference is due to chance is expressed as the *p value.* A *p* value of $<.05$ indicates there is less than a 5% chance that the difference observed could be due to chance alone.

It should be noted that if a difference is statistically significant, it may be real but not necessarily important. Or, the failure of an observed difference to achieve statistical significance may not mean that the difference is not real. Rather, it may indicate simply that the circumstances of the observation are such that a difference of the size observed could not be distinguished from the effects of chance alone.

Sampling and confidence intervals. To make a general observation about a population, it is customary to draw a sample from the population, make an observation based on the sample, and infer that the result applies to the population. For this technique to work, precautions must be taken to ensure that the sample is representative of the population. One way to do this is *randomization* of the sample, which means that each person in the population has an equal chance of being in the sample. Even with perfect randomization, the result found in one sample will likely differ from the result in a separate, similar sample. This is due to chance variation from one sample to the next. Given an observation from one sample, such as a measured average, it is possible to statistically compute the range around the average observed in the sample within which the true average of the population lies. This is referred to as a *confidence interval*. The confidence interval is specifically computed at some level of proba-bility, for example 90% or 95%. Thus, for a 95% confidence interval, there is a 95% likelihood that the true population average will lie within it, and a 5% likelihood that the true average will lie outside. In survey work (e.g., opinion polling), the proportion of persons in a representative sample with a specific response is determined. This proportion is often expressed with a confidence interval, showing the range within which the population's value is likely to lie. The width of a confidence interval increases when the degree of confidence is raised. Thus a 95% confidence interval is wider than one at 90%.

Additional Reading

Friedman, G. D. (1994). *Primer of epidemiology* (4th ed.). New York: McGraw-Hill. (See chapters 2 and 3.)

Hill, A. B. (1965). *Principles of medical statistics* (9th ed.). New York: Oxford.

Last, J. M. (1995). *A dictionary of epidemiology* (3rd ed.). New York: Oxford.

Lilienfeld, D. E., & Stolley, P. D. (1994). *Foundations of epidemiology* (3rd ed.). New York: Oxford. (See chapters 4-6.)

Norman. G., & Streiner, D. (1994). *Biostatistics: The bare essentials*. St. Louis, MO: Mosby.

Chapter 6

Making Inferences
From Observations

This chapter reviews some of the ways epidemiologists try to establish that a possible determinant for a disease is actually a determinant and not merely coincidental. Understanding causal association is obviously important if preventive strategies are to be developed. Presumed causal associations are frequently reported in the press and elsewhere. Knowing how to interpret claims of causal association requires an ability to evaluate the methods used. It is important to have some understanding of the various techniques used to evaluate possible associations and appreciate the value and limitations of each. Creutzfeldt-Jakob disease in Great Britain, which broke into the public press as well as the public health journals in 1996, is an example.

Creutzfeldt-Jakob disease (CJD) is a rare but devastating neurologic disease. It results in death in less than a year after onset of symptoms. It is transmissible under certain circumstances. CJD shares characteristics of conditions that have been found in sheep and cattle, including bovine spongiform encephalopathy (BSE), or "mad cow disease." This, plus aspects of the pathology noted in the brain suggest that it is due to a type of transmissible agent called a prion.[1] Emergence of what seemed to be a variant of CJD in Great Britain, affecting initially 10 young people and running a particularly rapid course (Will et al., 1996), raised concerns that BSE may be transmitted from cattle to humans and concerns that it could be occurring elsewhere (Centers for Disease Control and Prevention [CDC], 1996c). The observed association resulted in a sudden and dramatic decline in the market for beef products from Great Britain, and steps were taken to exterminate cattle herds. Decisions having great economic effect were made under tremendous political pressure. Are animals with BSE truly the source of CJD? To say the least, it is important to examine the validity of any inference of causality in the observed association of diseases in humans and in cattle.

It is the job of the epidemiologist to identify the associations related to a condition and tease apart those that may be causal from those that result from methodological *bias,* or from *confounding,* or are only coincidentally associated. *Hypotheses,* proposed explanations about cause, need to be tested. Often this is a complicated and difficult task. The ability to disentangle with confidence the causal from confounding variables depends in part on the strength of the epidemiological methods used by the epidemiologist. This chapter describes these methods of observation. Once a causal association is established, further exploration is often needed to understand the biological, behavioral, and social mechanisms of host interaction to design effective preventive interventions.

Two major categories of research are used to systematically test a hypothesis about causal association: observational and experimental studies. In observational studies, the epidemiologist obtains information from occurrences that have taken place. Ultimately observational studies are limited in allowing definitive conclusions about causation. In experimental studies, or *controlled interventions (clinical trials),* the investigator sets up and controls the variables being studied. The principal types of observational and experimental studies are briefly described here.

Ecological Studies

Ecological studies are observations about occurrences of a disease within populations where the disease is noted to be temporally associated with some phenomenon or exposure in the same population. The exposure is then posed as a possible cause. With ecological observations, there is no determination of whether the specific individuals who have the condition had greater exposure to the hypothesized causal variable than individuals without the condition. Rather, overall incidence rates for the condition are correlated with the occurrence rates of the proposed exposure.

The association of BSE with CJD, as described previously, is an example of an ecological association. What was observed was the persistent presence of BSE in cattle in Great Britain concurrent with the apparent increase in CJD in people in Great Britain. The initial analysis determined that the changing rates for both were temporally associated. There was a greater incidence of CJD where spongiform encephalopathy was prevalent (that is, in Great Britain), and a lessor incidence of CJD when BSE was rare or absent (such as elsewhere in Europe and in North America). Ecological associations, assuming the original observations are verified, are very useful in generating hypotheses about causation. They do not, however, establish that the observed relationship is causal. It may simply be coincidental that both are occurring in association, or each may be occurring as a result of some other common cause that is not yet apparent, and they would not be themselves causally tied to one another. The ecological fallacy occurs when an investigator infers causality in the face of coincidental association.

Case Reports

Like ecological observations, *case reports* are strictly descriptive. In a case report, the exposure and the outcome are observed to be linked in a few people, or even in only one person. The case report is useful in raising a causal hypothesis or in supporting an existing hypothesis.

Case reports have been very important in directing epidemiologists to further studies leading to additional investigation that can establish causal factors.

An example of a case report was the observed association of angiosarcoma (a type of cancer) of the liver in workers with occupational exposure to vinyl chloride (CDC, 1997b). Even when the case report seems to link an event with subsequent disease, it cannot alone distinguish causal association from coincidental association. Additional studies were needed to confirm the association of cancer with vinyl chloride.

Cross-Sectional Studies

Cross-sectional studies are typically the product of a sample survey of a population. It is a cross section because it looks at the population at a moment in time. In this sense, it is a tabulation of prevalence. The prevalence of any single observed variable can be directly computed. More important, the data can be analyzed for association of multiple variables within individuals in the population, making cross-sectional studies intrinsically stronger than ecological studies. They are stronger than case reports because there is an opportunity to quantitatively examine the rates of association of a presumed exposure in persons with a health condition and in those without the condition. As a descriptive approach, cross-sectional studies can establish association and support hypotheses, but cannot clearly distinguish causality.

Prospective Cohort Studies

The *prospective cohort study* can be of enormous value in identifying associations and in generating and refining hypotheses. A key feature is that the study groups, or *cohorts*, are followed forward in time to watch for the emergence of the health outcome of interest. An important advantage of this method of epidemiologic observation is that incidences may be computed and compared and relative risks calcu-

TABLE 6.1　Schema for Analysis of a Prospective Cohort Study

	Group With Exposure	Group Without Exposure
Disease occurs	a	b
No disease occurs	c	d
	a + c	b + d

Incidence in the group with exposure: a / (a + c)
Incidence in the group without exposure: b / (b + d)
Relative risk of the exposure: (a / (a + b)) / (b / (b + d))

lated (see Table 6.1). A classification by exposure is done using data gathered before the outcome has occurred. This is an advantage over *retrospective studies*, those that look backward in time, in that recall and selection biases are minimized. Recall bias may be introduced when either the investigator or the subject has knowledge of the outcome at the time when information about the exposure is collected. Selection bias occurs when a study sample is selected in such a way that there is an association with the exposure variable as a part of the sampling process itself.

In prospective cohort studies, one cohort that has received exposure to the hypothesized agent or factor is compared with another cohort without the exposure. The lack of control over exposure may result in erroneous conclusions about causation. Even when the exposure is shown to be associated with a disease, the association may not be causal. There may in fact be some additional, unsuspected factor of causal significance with which the hypothesized "causal" factor is somehow associated. This interaction of factors is called *confounding*.

A practical disadvantage of prospective designs is that the cohorts must be followed over time. If there is prolonged latency, that is, the time between exposure and clinically detectable outcome, the time required for follow-up can make such studies burdensome. For some outcomes, such as cancer, latencies will be measured in years or even decades. Also, because the incidence rates are often low, it is usually necessary to follow large numbers, sometimes thousands or even tens of thousands, of subjects in some cohort groups. The large number of subjects, the length of time, and the requirement for meticulous tracking and follow-up all make some prospective studies difficult and costly, with results that are unavailable for years.

The following are two examples of prospective cohort studies that have been of major public health importance. A follow-up of survivors of atomic blasts in 1945 in Japan, with careful sorting by estimated dose of exposure, has become the single most important source of information about dose-effects of radiation for cancers and birth anomalies. The second example, also begun in the 1940s, is a long-term study of men in Framingham, Massachusetts. This was the initial major longitudinal study that verified and permitted quantitative characterization of the association of effects of various risk factors on cardiovascular disease, including elevated blood cholesterol, high blood pressure, and smoking.

Case-Control Studies

Case-control studies have been a particularly useful tool for efficiently identifying factors associated with disease and other conditions of concern. In contrast with the prospective studies just described, case-control studies can be performed rapidly and require observations only on actual cases and a corresponding number of *controls,* or persons without the condition. Rather than starting with persons who have (or have not) been exposed to some possible risk and then awaiting an outcome, the case-control method goes directly to persons with the outcome. It then looks back in time to see what may have affected that outcome. Histories of exposure are taken from these cases and from the controls. The proportion of cases with the exposure is then compared with the corresponding proportion of controls having the same exposure (see Table 6.2). A statistically significant increased proportion in the cases compared with the controls suggests an association between the exposure and the disease. The case-control approach analyzes rather than simply describes the association of hypothesized exposure variables in persons with and without the disease.

TABLE 6.2 Schema for Analysis of Case-Control Study

	Cases	Controls
History of exposure	a	b
No history of exposure	c	d
	a + c	b + d

Proportion of all cases who were exposed: a / (a + c)
Proportion of all controls who were exposed: b / (b + d)
If the exposure contributed to the disease, the proportion of cases who were exposed will be greater than the proportion of controls who were exposed.
Odds ratio: (a × d) / (b × c)[1]

NOTE: 1. The odds ratio is computed in case-control studies in place of a relative risk. The derivation of the formula shown for the odds ratio depends on certain conditions being met and goes beyond the scope of this book.

There are limitations and pitfalls in conducting case-control studies. First, the investigator does not have the opportunity to observe unanticipated outcomes for a given exposure. Rather, only one specific outcome is explored by virtue of cases being the point of entry. Obviously, the cause must be already suspected so that it can be specifically sought in gathering the histories from the cases and controls. Second, incidence rates and relative risks cannot be directly measured because only the cases and their controls are entered into the analysis. The population from which they come is not considered. Relative risk may be approximated in many instances by calculating the relative odds or *odds ratio*. Third, if the control group is not similar in its characteristics to the cases in every way (other than the exposure), differences in proportions exposed may be misleading due to introduction of confounding variables. Fourth, there are opportunities for bias at several points. For example, the process of selecting cases (or controls) may inadvertently include persons who have disproportionately been subjected to the hypothesized exposure. Or, persons who are cases may be motivated to recall past events in greater detail than someone who is a healthy control. These are examples, respectively, of selection and recall biases. Because of such pitfalls, the investigating epidemiologist must use caution. It is helpful to be able to have multiple studies confirming the same hypothesis.

Because of their relative efficiency and low cost, case-control studies have been widely used. They are very common in analyzing risk factors for chronic disease such as cancers and vascular disease. Case-control studies may help clarify the hypothesized linkage between BSE and CJD.

Case-control methods are also used in acute outbreaks of illness to identify or implicate a specific source of exposure. For example, in seeking the specific contaminated food item in an illness emanating from a source such as a restaurant, the public health epidemiologist will compare food items ingested by those who became ill (cases) with food items ingested by those who did not (controls). Often the offending item can be rapidly and precisely identified.

Controlled Interventions

The *controlled intervention* is a special type of prospective cohort study. It follows prospectively groups (cohorts) that have and have not been subject to some sort of exposure or intervention. What makes controlled interventions special is that the exposure or intervention is controlled by the investigator, instead of simply occurring in the course of the subjects' lives. That is, the investigator determines who gets the exposure or intervention and who does not. In this respect, the controlled intervention is a planned experiment.

The ability to control the exposure provides important advantages over observational approaches such as the prospective cohort study. By carefully randomizing the subjects into exposure and control categories, every variable other than the exposure will tend to be equalized across the comparison groups. This greatly reduces the possibility of confounding. Furthermore, it is often possible to disguise who gets the exposure in such a way that the subject will not be aware of which group (exposure or control) he or she is in, and thereby will not be biased in reporting outcomes. This is a *blinded study*. Use of *placebos* and sham exposure can be helpful in effectively "blinding" the subjects by disguising who may be in the control group. By use of coding, even the investigator can be blinded with respect to who has received the exposure, thereby reducing any bias in interpreting outcomes. Of course, the designations are eventually decoded for analysis. When both the subject and the investigator are blinded, it is a "double-blind" study.

The strength of the controlled intervention is that just one variable can be manipulated and analyzed. If the intervention produces an effect not seen in the control group, support will be given to any causal hypothesis that is tied to that intervention variable. Controlled interventions constitute the best source of information about the *efficacy* of a preventive maneuver or treatment. Examples include the determination of efficacy of immunization in preventing infection and the efficacy of antihypertensive medicines in reducing mortality from stroke and heart attacks in people with high blood pressure. Like the prospective cohort study, the controlled intervention takes time and can be expensive to conduct.

There are ethical issues that may arise in intervention studies, such as assigning persons to receive an exposure that could be harmful or assigning persons to treatment and control groups when the treatment may either be beneficial or, as sometimes happens, turn out to be worse than no treatment. For these reasons, intervention studies should be conducted only when there are real uncertainties about the efficacy of the intervention. On the other hand, rigorously controlled interventions may be the only way to determine efficacy. To proceed with a health-related intervention without the support of data from a controlled trial may itself be irresponsible or even reckless. The history of medicine and public health is strewn with the wreckage of well-accepted interventions that were later proved to have been unnecessary or ineffective after carefully controlled trials were done—for example, routine x-ray screening for lung cancer.

From the foregoing sections, it should be clear that epidemiological investigations can be difficult, have pitfalls that result in misleading conclusions, and, depending on the methods used, may be inherently limited in the extent to which causal inference can be made at all. Often what one has is only a hypothesis.

Epidemiological studies, well conducted and appropriately interpreted, provide the science on which public health decisions and policy must draw. Without good epidemiological foundations, public health would have only intuition and opinion to draw on.

It is reasonable and important to ask the question, when is causality actually determined? Most epidemiologists concur that, in general, one cannot absolutely prove something to be a cause. Nevertheless, a causal relationship can be established to the extent that causal inference can be made beyond any reasonable doubt. This will be achieved to the extent that the following criteria can be demonstrated: (a) consistency of the association, where the association is reproduced in a variety of settings; (b) strength of the association, where the effect is produced in the presence of the association and minimal or absent without the association occurring; (c) gradient of biological effect, where increasing the exposure results in increasing response; (d) temporality with the effect following the exposure and not simply being concurrent; (e) plausibility, where the effect is consistent with or can be explained in terms of existing science; (f) coherence in the body of evidence, where various separate lines of evidence are consistent; (g) experimental evidence confirms the association; and there are analogies with causal associations found in other settings (Hill, 1965, pp. 309-323; U.S. Department of Health, Education, and Welfare, 1964).

The criteria listed here were refined in response to the need to address whether smoking tobacco causes lung cancers. For tobacco, each of the criteria have been addressed. Establishing causal association does not have to mean that the causal mechanism is fully understood. That there is still research to be done, on what it is about tobacco smoke that causes cancer at the chemical and cellular levels and on why it is that not everyone gets cancer, does not invalidate the causal relationship between smoking and cancer. Of course, establishing a causal association does not exclude additional causes that result in the same outcome. Thus, lung cancer is caused by tobacco use and also by exposure to asbestos and radon.

Is BSE causally associated with CJD? One could not conclude causation based only on the initial ecological observation made in Great Britain. At that time, some measure of biological plausibility did exist, namely, features of prion infection. It would require either cohort or case-control analyses to establish that exposure to BSE actually occurred, preceding the disease, and to establish that risk increased with the extent of the exposure. The association would require consistent verification across multiple sets of observation. Cases of CJD not associated with BSE would have to be accounted for. One could not do a controlled intervention, but one would expect to see a decline in new cases following removal of sources of the hypothesized exposure.

Organized Research

The large-scale epidemiologic studies that have illuminated the determinants and risk factors for many illnesses (cancers, cardiovascular diseases, chronic pulmonary disease, HIV/AIDS, and many others) emerge in the context of federal prioritized research agendas and are funded through major public entities such as the National Institutes of Health, the Centers for Disease Control and Prevention, and large private foundations. The information gained is evaluated and adapted for public policies and interventions. It would be unusual for a local or even a state public health department to undertake such large-scale investigations. It is common and highly appropriate, however, for the local public health entity to undertake assessments of local outbreaks and of anomalously elevated rates of chronic or recurrent conditions. This is one of the core functions of a health department.

Even for the larger scale investigations, the point of initiation is often an astute observation by a local health officer or other person. As has been said, AIDS came to the world's attention on local recognition of a cluster of unusual tumors and infections among gay men. Other examples of recently recognized conditions include the discovery in the Southwest of what would later be characterized as hantavirus pulmonary syndrome by a physician who noted simultaneous cases of unexplained respiratory failure in two young adults (CDC, 1993). Another physician called local public health authorities' attention to a small cluster of cases of what would later be called eosinophilia-myalgia syndrome, a chronic, sometimes fatal illness that had been occurring but was unrecognized worldwide. Subsequent epidemiological analysis established that the syndrome was caused by ingestion of a manufactured preparation of tryptophan, an amino acid used as a sleep aid (Hertzman et al., 1990).

Cautionary Words

Epidemiological methods have proven to be enormously powerful tools in establishing the causal basis for disease. Effective public health strategies require this kind of information. It is essential, however, to avoid the error of overly focusing on one epidemiologically established cause when, in fact, there is in reality a web of causation, other components of which may hold the keys for effective public health intervention (see Chapter 4). The epidemiological methods reviewed in this chapter usually attempt to isolate a hypothesized elemental cause from its social environment. By controlling for variables that characterized such environments, environmental determinants are excluded from consideration. The web is cut away, and efforts at disease control may become misdirected. This may account for the ineffectiveness usually encountered in attempts to prevent chronic disease by urging people to alter behaviors epidemiologically proven to be tied with the disease. Although the behavior, such as a sedentary lifestyle, eating excessive dietary fats, and smoking, can be shown to be important, behavioral change interventions have generally poor records for long-term success. The underlying environmental issues that direct people toward such behaviors must also be addressed. The challenge for epidemiologists is to identify methods that will highlight the connectivity of variables within the causal web, or between the levels within the Chinese boxes (see Chapter 4), rather than simply isolate the causal variables.

Furthermore, simply knowing the causal pathway does not ensure that effective public health planning will follow. Although excellent scientific information is an important step for planning, it is only one component in the planning process. Planning is a complex interaction that involves, for example, political, economic, and social elements. This will be discussed further in Chapter 10.

Note

1. Prions are a class of transmissible agents that can cause disease. They are neither bacteria nor viruses, and do not contain genetic material. A prion is a protein, similar to a normal host protein, that uses the host protein as material to replicate itself inside a cell. If the new prion material accumulates without being removed by the cell, it will destroy the cell.

Additional Reading

Friedman, G. D. (1994). *Primer of epidemiology* (4th ed.). New York: McGraw-Hill. (See chapters 4-11.)

Lilienfeld, D. E., & Stolley, P. D. (1994). *Foundations of epidemiology* (3rd ed.). New York: Oxford. (See chapters 6-12.)

Chapter 7

Surveillance and Monitoring the Health of Populations

The preceding three chapters have provided overviews of how epidemiology is used to understand the determinants of disease and of the language used for some epidemiologic measures and methods. This chapter describes how epidemiology fits into the practice of public health. The topics covered fall within the assessment function of public health. Common sources of information are described. Additional topics include risk assessment and measurement of outcomes.

Surveillance and Monitoring

The bulk of day-to-day epidemiological activity done in public health practice involves surveillance and monitoring for known disease. *Surveillance* is the continuous search for and documentation of the rate of occurrence of a disease or condition. Surveillance involves analysis and interpretation of the data and dissemination to those who need to know (Centers for Disease Control and Prevention, 1986). Surveillance is done to achieve early detection of outbreaks and institute a timely response. In some instances, identification of even a single case will be of importance. This occurs when even one case of an otherwise infrequent or rare infection could result in rapid spread by person-to-person contact in a susceptible population. Examples include measles, meningococcal meningitis, and tuberculosis. Some conditions are important because they may indicate a single source of infection or toxic exposure that could threaten others, such as cholera and hepatitis A from water supplies, *Escherichia coli* and salmonella from food sources, and pesticide and lead poisoning from an occupational or other environmental source. A condition for which a single case is enough to initiate an immediate investigation because an occurrence implies a breakdown of normal preventive controls is called a *sentinel condition* (Rutstein et al., 1976).

For other conditions that are expected to occur in the population with a measure of predictability, it is important to monitor for changes in incidence rates. *Monitoring* is the routine measurement of the status of occurrence of such diseases to detect changes in the environment or in effectiveness of prevention and control measures. Most diseases for which immunizations are available are monitored. Figure 7.1 shows results of monitoring incidence of invasive *Haemophilus influenzae* type b infection in children in selected cities in the United States. This agent had been the leading cause of meningitis in children until a vaccine was introduced and achieved widespread use in the late 1980s. Monitoring clearly documents the effectiveness of the vaccine.

Also monitored are levels of environmental pollution or contamination. In addition, public health concerns itself with managing risks for many chronic conditions. Cardiovascular diseases, cancers, cirrhosis of the liver, congenital anomalies, and complications of diabetes are among the chronic conditions that are monitored.

To track deaths, infectious diseases, toxic effects, injuries, and chronic conditions, effective surveillance and monitoring systems are needed. The development and maintenance of valid monitoring systems are among the most important assessment tasks of public health.

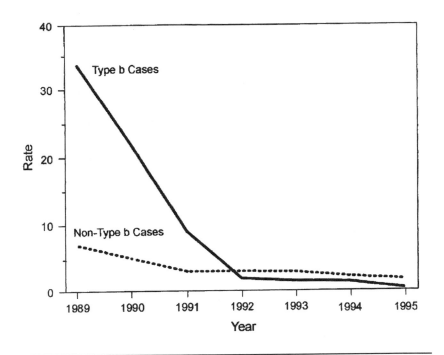

Figure 7.1. Race-Adjusted Incidence Rate for Invasive *Haemophilus influenzae* Type B and Non-Type B Disease Among Children Aged <5 Years, in the United States, 1989-1995
SOURCE: Centers for Disease Control and Prevention (1996e).
NOTE: Per 100,000 children aged <5 years.

Sources of Information

Vital records. Vital records, birth certificates and death certificates (see Figure 7.2) occupy a central position in information gathering. Birth and death certificates are required by law in every state. Birth certificates are the source of data for measures of prenatal care and health such as birth weight, gestational age, when prenatal care was started, information about congenital defects observable at birth, and information about the mother such as age and residence. In addition to providing information about infant health, such information is an important component needed to determine fertility rates and estimate population growth rates. Death certificates are the single most important and most extensively used source of information regarding causes

U.S. STANDARD
CERTIFICATE OF DEATH

TYPE/PRINT
IN
PERMANENT
BLACK INK
FOR
INSTRUCTIONS

SEE OTHER SIDE
AND HANDBOOK

LOCAL FILE NUMBER | STATE FILE NUMBER

1. DECEDENT'S NAME (First, Middle, Last): John Leonard Palmer

2. SEX: Male
3. DATE OF DEATH (Month, Day, Year): June 20, 1989

4. SOCIAL SECURITY NUMBER: 123-45-6789
5a. AGE—Last Birthday (Years): 78
5b. UNDER 1 YEAR — Months | Days
5c. UNDER 1 DAY — Hours | Minutes
6. DATE OF BIRTH (Month, Day, Year): April 23, 1911
7. BIRTHPLACE (City and State or Foreign Country): San Francisco, CA

8. WAS DECEDENT EVER IN U.S. ARMED FORCES? (Yes or no): Yes

9a. PLACE OF DEATH (Check only one, see instructions on other side)
HOSPITAL: ☒ Inpatient ☐ ER/Outpatient ☐ DOA
OTHER: ☐ Nursing Home ☐ Residence ☐ Other (Specify)

9b. FACILITY NAME (If not institution give street and number): Mountain Memorial Hospital
9c. CITY, TOWN, OR LOCATION OF DEATH: Frederick
9d. COUNTY OF DEATH: Frederick

10. MARITAL STATUS — Married ☐ Never Married ☐ Widowed ☐ Divorced (Specify): Married
11. SURVIVING SPOUSE (If wife, give maiden name): Sheila Marie Sonner

12a. DECEDENT'S USUAL OCCUPATION (Give kind of work done during most of working life. Do not use retired): Certified Public Accountant
12b. KIND OF BUSINESS/INDUSTRY: Self-employed

13a. RESIDENCE STATE: Maryland
13b. COUNTY: Frederick
13c. CITY, TOWN, OR LOCATION: Thurmont
13d. STREET AND NUMBER: 245 Lone View Road

13e. INSIDE CITY LIMITS? (Yes or no): No
13f. ZIP CODE: 20212

14. WAS DECEDENT OF HISPANIC ORIGIN? (Specify No or Yes. If yes specify Cuban, Mexican, Puerto Rican etc.): ☒ No — Specify
15. RACE—American Indian, Black, White, etc. (Specify): White
16. DECEDENT'S EDUCATION (Specify only highest grade completed) Elementary/Secondary (0-12) | College (1-4 or 5+): 4

17. FATHER'S NAME (First, Middle, Last): Stanley Leonard Palmer
18. MOTHER'S NAME (First, Middle, Maiden Surname): Lorraine Ellen Russell

19a. INFORMANT'S NAME (Type/Print): Sheila Marie Palmer
19b. MAILING ADDRESS (Street and Number or Rural Route Number, City or Town, State, Zip Code): 245 Lone View Road, Thurmont, MD 20212

20a. METHOD OF DISPOSITION
☒ Burial ☐ Cremation ☐ Removal from State
☐ Donation ☐ Other (Specify)

20b. PLACE OF DISPOSITION (Name of cemetery, crematory, or other place): Wesley Memorial Cemetery
20c. LOCATION—City or Town, State: Frederick, MD

21a. SIGNATURE OF FUNERAL SERVICE LICENSEE OR PERSON ACTING AS SUCH: Robert J. Boone
21b. LICENSE NUMBER (of Licensee): 2569114
22. NAME AND ADDRESS OF FACILITY: Boone and Sons Funeral Home 475 E. Main St., Frederick, MD 20216

23a. To the best of my knowledge, death occurred at the time, date, and place stated.
Signature and Title ▶ Julia D. Kovac, M.D.
23b. LICENSE NUMBER: 62499075
23c. DATE SIGNED (Month, Day, Year): June 20, 1989

24. TIME OF DEATH
25. DATE PRONOUNCED DEAD (Month, Day, Year)
26. WAS CASE REFERRED TO MEDICAL EXAMINER/CORONER?

Complete items 23a-c only when certifying physician is not available at time of death to certify cause of death

SEE DEFINITION ON OTHER SIDE

ITEMS 24-26 MUST BE COMPLETED BY PERSON WHO

NAME OF DECEDENT
SEE INSTRUCTIONS ON OTHER SIDE
For use by physician or institution

J. LEONARD PALMER

CENTER FOR HEALTH STATISTICS - 1989 REVISION

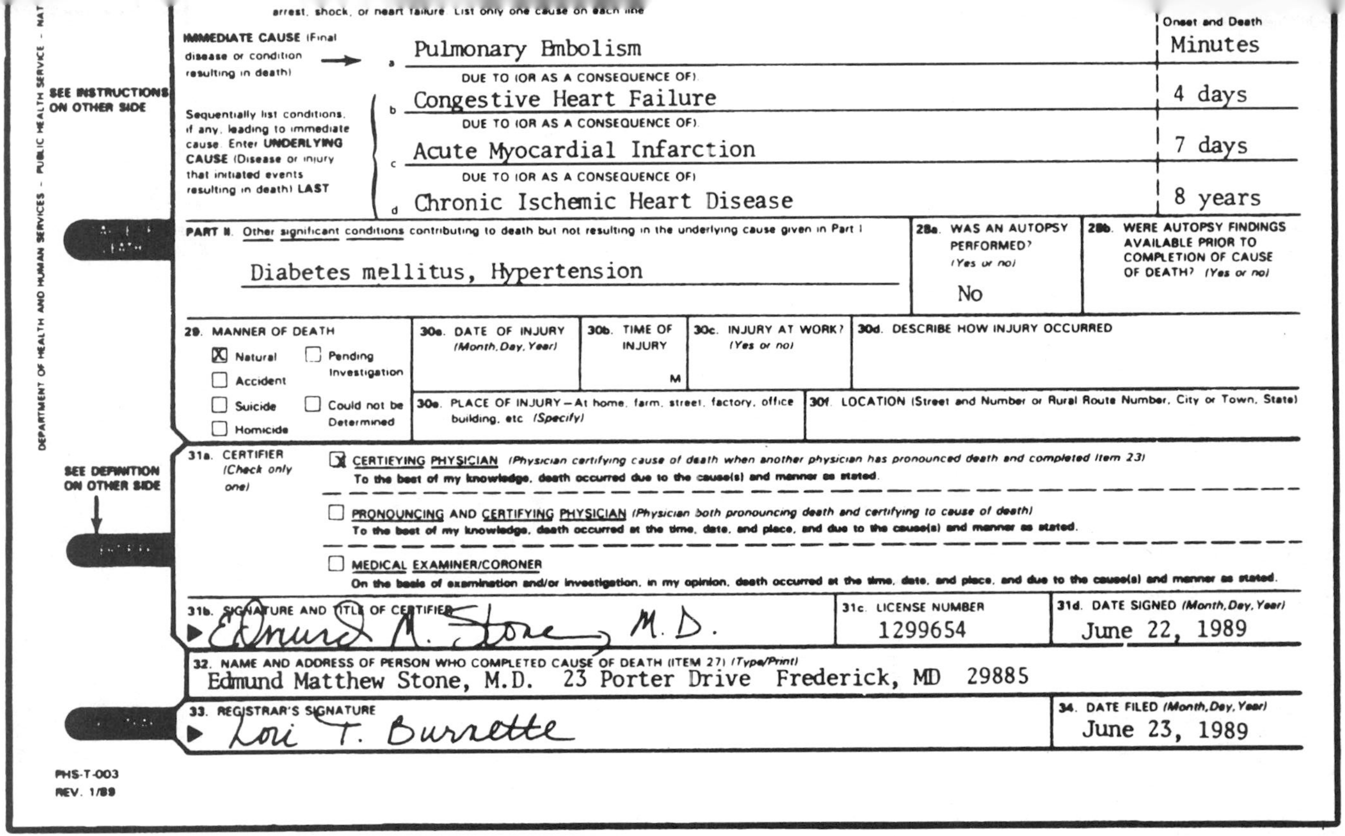

arrest, shock, or heart failure. List only one cause on each line

DEPARTMENT OF HEALTH AND HUMAN SERVICES - PUBLIC HEALTH SERVICE - NAT

SEE INSTRUCTIONS ON OTHER SIDE

			Onset and Death
IMMEDIATE CAUSE (Final disease or condition resulting in death) →	a	Pulmonary Embolism	Minutes
		DUE TO (OR AS A CONSEQUENCE OF):	
Sequentially list conditions, if any, leading to immediate cause. Enter UNDERLYING CAUSE (Disease or injury that initiated events resulting in death) LAST	b	Congestive Heart Failure	4 days
		DUE TO (OR AS A CONSEQUENCE OF):	
	c	Acute Myocardial Infarction	7 days
		DUE TO (OR AS A CONSEQUENCE OF):	
	d	Chronic Ischemic Heart Disease	8 years

PART II. Other significant conditions contributing to death but not resulting in the underlying cause given in Part I

Diabetes mellitus, Hypertension

28a. WAS AN AUTOPSY PERFORMED? (Yes or no) No

28b. WERE AUTOPSY FINDINGS AVAILABLE PRIOR TO COMPLETION OF CAUSE OF DEATH? (Yes or no)

29. MANNER OF DEATH

- [x] Natural
- [ ] Accident
- [ ] Suicide
- [ ] Homicide
- [ ] Pending Investigation
- [ ] Could not be Determined

30a. DATE OF INJURY (Month, Day, Year)

30b. TIME OF INJURY M

30c. INJURY AT WORK? (Yes or no)

30d. DESCRIBE HOW INJURY OCCURRED

30e. PLACE OF INJURY—At home, farm, street, factory, office building, etc. (Specify)

30f. LOCATION (Street and Number or Rural Route Number, City or Town, State)

SEE DEFINITION ON OTHER SIDE

31a. CERTIFIER (Check only one)

- [x] CERTIFYING PHYSICIAN (Physician certifying cause of death when another physician has pronounced death and completed Item 23) To the best of my knowledge, death occurred due to the cause(s) and manner as stated.
- [ ] PRONOUNCING AND CERTIFYING PHYSICIAN (Physician both pronouncing death and certifying to cause of death) To the best of my knowledge, death occurred at the time, date, and place, and due to the cause(s) and manner as stated.
- [ ] MEDICAL EXAMINER/CORONER On the basis of examination and/or investigation, in my opinion, death occurred at the time, date, and place, and due to the cause(s) and manner as stated.

31b. SIGNATURE AND TITLE OF CERTIFIER ▶ Edmund M. Stone, M.D.

31c. LICENSE NUMBER 1299654

31d. DATE SIGNED (Month, Day, Year) June 22, 1989

32. NAME AND ADDRESS OF PERSON WHO COMPLETED CAUSE OF DEATH (ITEM 27) (Type/Print)
Edmund Matthew Stone, M.D. 23 Porter Drive Frederick, MD 29885

33. REGISTRAR'S SIGNATURE ▶ Lori T. Burnette

34. DATE FILED (Month, Day, Year) June 23, 1989

PHS-T-003
REV. 1/89

Figure 7.2. Death Certificate

SOURCE: U.S. Department of Health and Human Services. (1988). *Guidelines for reporting occupation and industry on death certificates.* (p. 29). (DHHS Publication No. [PHS] 88-1149). Hyattsville, MD: Author.

of death. The information is tabulated in a standardized manner by state vital records departments and forwarded for collation to the National Center for Health Statistics at the Centers for Disease Control and Prevention (CDC). The usefulness of the information depends on its accuracy. It is sometimes unclear what causes a death. Relevant underlying or co-morbid conditions may be overlooked or underreported. Mortality statistics are of no use regarding conditions that are not lethal. They do not reflect morbidity and disability from chronic conditions that are either nonfatal or fatal only after a long period.

Reportable conditions. State law requires the reporting of certain conditions of public health importance, most notably, infectious diseases, to the health department. Data are analyzed for evidence of general changes in incidence, outbreaks, and breaches in the systems of prevention and control. Reporting is required of medical providers and of laboratories where microbial pathogens are isolated or serologic testing is done. The states send the information to the CDC, where it is collated for the country (see Table 7.1).

Other health conditions are reported through other systems. Pesticide poisoning must be reported in some states. Child abuse and other abuses must be reported to the appropriate state agency. Occupational injuries and deaths must be reported to the federal or state *Occupational Safety and Health Administration (OSHA)*. Motor vehicle crashes are reported to highway traffic and safety authorities.

Surveys. Surveys are very useful ways of obtaining information about people's health in general, about chronic conditions, and other things such as health-related behaviors. Such information will, of course, not be available in vital records. The National Center for Health Statistics conducts several ongoing surveys that provide very important information. Careful selection of the survey samples and high rates of participation permit statistical extrapolation to the general population. The National Health Interview Survey and the National Health and Nutrition Examination Survey are two examples.

Developed and supported by the CDC, the Behavioral Risk Factor Sample Survey is a telephone survey of adults, conducted in most

TABLE 7.1 Infectious Diseases Designated as Notifiable—United States, 1996

Acquired immunodeficiency syndrome	Legionellosis
Anthrax	Lyme disease
Botulism	Malaria
Brucellosis	Measles
Chancroid	Meningococcal disease
Chlamydia trachomatis, genital infection	Mumps
Cholera	Pertussis
Coccidioidomycosis	Plague
Congenital rubella syndrome	Poliomyelitis, paralytic
Congenital syphilis	Psittacosis
Cryptosporidiosis	Rabies, animal
Diphtheria	Rabies, human
Encephalitis, California	Rocky Mountain spotted fever
Encephalitis, eastern equine	Rubella
Encephalitis, St. Louis	Salmonellosis
Encephalitis, western equine	Shigellosis
Escherichia coli 0157:H7	Streptococcal disease, invasive, group A
Gonorrhea	
Haemophilus influenzae, invasive disease	*Streptococcus pneumoniae*, drug-resistant
Hansens's disease (Leprosy)	Streptococcal toxic shock syndrome
Hantavirus pulmonary syndrome	Syphilis
Hemolytic uremic syndrome, postdiarrheal	Tetanus
	Toxic shock syndrome
Hepatitis A	Trichinosis
Hepatitis B	Tuberculosis
Hepatitis C/non-A, non-B	Typhoid fever
HIV infection, pediatric	Yellow fever

SOURCE: Centers for Disease Control and Prevention (1996d, p. 42).

states, using nationally standardized protocols. It tabulates the prevalence of individual risk factors. The CDC also has supported the state-based Youth Risk Behavior Surveillance System monitoring health risk behaviors in high school students. Prevalence rates may be traced over time. Although generally useful for examining statewide trends, data from these statewide surveys will not necessarily clarify a local situation or health need. Supplementary local assessments, including more specific and targeted surveys, may need to be conducted. Surveys are labor intensive and generally costly to administer.

Hospital discharge data. Most states require the reporting of hospital discharge information, including inpatient discharge diagnosis. This allows tabulation of illness events. Interpretation of the data and usefulness for tracking disease rates are problematic to the extent that patterns of use of hospitals for illnesses vary by region and change over time. Furthermore, multiple admissions for the same illness can occur. Alternatively, as people become enrolled in managed care systems that supply all or most of their care, administrative databases should be able to link information about individuals, their illness events, and chronic disease diagnoses. It should be possible to use such databases and information systems in the future for public health purposes, including tracking morbidity and identifying sentinel events and patterns of outbreaks.

Registries. Registries attempt to identify all cases of a specified condition occurring within a defined geographic area. This is of greatest help for those conditions that are not otherwise reported, or that would not be adequately characterized through death reports, for which there is particular concern about changing incidences. For example, the National Cancer Institute supports a set of tumor registries representing various regions and population groups around the United States. Working with providers, hospitals, and pathology laboratories, an effort is made to record and follow all recognized cases of cancer. This has proven to be an excellent way to track the incidence of cancer over time.

Defining the Population

Except for sentinel conditions, where the occurrence of one case is enough to act on, counts of death and disease must be expressed in terms of the population. That is, new cases are expressed as incidence rates. Deaths are expressed as mortality rates. Survey data are expressed as proportions in a population. Moreover, such rates often will have to be adjusted for age, sex, and sometimes other elements in the population profile. Without these steps, a count of events at any one time cannot be compared with other counts over time within the same population or across different populations. This is because populations differ and change with time. It is, thus, crucial to have an accurate characterization of the population being observed, that is, numbers in the population by age, sex, and racial group. This information on populations is provided by the national census. Census information, however, is gathered only every 10 years. It undercounts some groups that are of particular public health importance such as the homeless, undocumented aliens, and certain minority groups. More important, changes in some of these population groups can occur rapidly due to migrations. All of these factors need to be taken into account by the public health epidemiologist.

Risk Assessment and Communication

In addition to identifying the causal basis for disease, the epidemiologist must also assess the importance of risks and communicate this information to the public. Risk assessment is based on studies of incidence following exposure, and using information about relative risk to calculate an estimation of attributable risk (see Chapters 4, 5, and 6).

Public perception of risk often does not match the epidemiologic assessment of risk, and people may not be persuaded by evidence. Some situations with relatively high risk may be ignored, whereas other situations with extraordinarily low risk are considered unacceptable by the public. Examples include tolerance of unsafe automobiles and intolerance to threat of exposure to radiation levels too low to register measurable individual risk. Perception of risk is influenced by many factors. Among these are the extent to which a condition is unfamiliar, the extent to which the risk is perceived with fear and dread, and the extent to which people feel they have no control. Perception of risk increases when people feel they cannot trust sources of information such as governmental authorities, manufacturers, or the media (Slovic, 1987).

Perceptions that exaggerate risk may lead to dramatic and costly actions with very uncertain benefit. For example, several common rheumatologic conditions were attributed to effects of silicone breast implants, but without any consistent epidemiologic evidence to support this assertion. This resulted in lawsuits with billions of dollars in settlements and in corporate bankruptcy (Angell, 1996). In 1989, information was aired on television that Alar, a growth regulator that had been routinely sprayed on apples since 1968, caused cancer in humans. Apple sales immediately plummeted, with losses to producers of hundreds of millions of dollars. The source of the information was data from research conducted in 1977 on mice exposed to massive amounts of the chemical. This research had previously been viewed by the EPA as flawed and unsuitable for assessing risk for cancer in humans. The FDA, WHO, and other authorities continue to stress that Alar is not a risk to public health (Reynolds, n.d.).

Risk assessment and risk management are essential elements in development of public health policy that regulates hazards in the environment (Ruckelshaus, 1983). In practice, however, the public policy that regulates those hazards emerges from a negotiated process involving multiple participants, each with a perception of the risk and each with a stake in the outcome. Scientific assessment of risk is but one of the inputs in this process. The challenge for the public health provider who is trying to communicate information about risk is to find a balance that, while accurately conveying what is known about a risk, must also remain sensitive to the reality of public perception.

Outcomes and Effectiveness

Efficacy and effectiveness. An important aspect of public health surveillance is the need to document the *effectiveness* of interventions taken. Effectiveness is not the same as *efficacy*. Information about efficacy is developed in carefully controlled investigational settings where various compliance conditions are met. Determination of efficacy is critically important because it indicates what can be done. In putting the information into practice in the field, however, there is no assurance that the full potential reflected in efficacy studies will be realized. That is to say, the intervention may be efficacious, but not effective. Effectiveness refers to the extent to which the intervention works when it is attempted under field conditions. For example, a vaccine may be tested as being 90% efficacious in preventing an infectious disease and be less than 50% effective in the population in which it is used. There can be many reasons for this: improper storage with loss of potency, improper administration technique, differences in responsiveness in the target population compared with the test population, and refusal of the population to accept the vaccine. Assessment of outcomes is always important until effectiveness is demonstrated. Unfortunately, too many public health efforts neglect this crucial step.

Measures of Overall Health

Monitoring is most often conducted in the context of specific diseases or conditions. Tracking individual diseases, however, does not provide a picture of the general health of the population. Agencies and governing bodies that have responsibility for the health of the public or interest in value for the money spent are seeking accountability for improvements in general health. Can health be documented? Can the general health status of one population be compared with that of others?

The technology for monitoring overall health is incompletely developed, whether one is measuring the health of individuals or the aggregate health of a population. Instruments to measure the functional status of individuals and quality of life are in use, for example, the short-form health survey (SF-36) (Ware & Sherbourne, 1992). These questionnaires are cumbersome and costly to administer to general populations. The full range of their usefulness is the subject of current research (Testa & Simonson, 1996). The CDC has introduced questions that ask about one's general physical and mental health in the Behavioral Risk Factor Survey. Such measures, gathered across a population sample, may be used to generate an index of a population's health. Another approach, presently being explored by the Institute of Medicine and others, is to assemble a composite indicator from available measures of mortality, incidences of preventable disease, and prevalences of health risk behaviors. Each of these approaches continues to be hampered, however, in that there is no agreed-on method for measuring health as a positive condition, as opposed to the absence of disease.

Additional Reading

Gotsch, A. R., & Goldstein, B. (Eds.). (1996). Communicating environmental risk to the public [Special issue]. *Health Education Quarterly, 18*(3).

Part III

PUBLIC HEALTH INTERVENTIONS
AND APPLICATIONS

The chapters in the previous section have presented an overview of the epidemiology of assessment—tools that are used to compile and analyze health data, generate understanding of the conditions that determine health status, and allow health program planning to proceed scientifically, grounded on evidence. Without the analytic tools, the rational development of policies and programs to address health problems could not exist. The chapters in this section introduce basic approaches used in public health intervention: health promotion and health protection (Chapter 8), personal health care services within public health (Chapter 9), and health planning (Chapter 10).

Public health practice ranges across a continuum from local initiatives on behalf of individuals to the global initiatives that can impact the health of millions of people. Chapter 11 focuses on the latter end of this continuum. It examines some of the issues that affect the health of the world's nearly 6 billion inhabitants and the approaches taken through internationally based initiatives to address them. The chapter draws on the basic principles of health and disease, understanding of determinants, and approaches to intervention that have been laid out in the preceding sections. Among the lessons that emerge with respect to global public health is that for international health strategies to be accepted and effective, they eventually must incorporate individual and community participation at regional and local levels.

Chapter 8

Health Promotion
and Health Protection

The prevention of disease and the promotion of good health are among the most basic goals of public health. This chapter will present an overview of the concept of health promotion and health protection. Chapter 9 will examine the role of prevention in personal health care services.

The Concept of Health Promotion

The Emerging Importance of Individual Lifestyle in Health

Over the years, as infectious disease was diminishing and chronic disease was increasing as the major cause of human mortality, the approach to disease control changed. In the decades that followed

World War II, the burden of chronic disease and the limitations and costs of medical management were increasingly apparent. The causes of chronic disease were multifactorial. Long-term epidemiological studies such as the Framingham Study of coronary heart disease pointed to personal risk factors that were influenced by the behavior of the individual as contributors to the susceptibility to that disease. Public health efforts in disease control evolved from a primary focus on the avoidance of communicable disease toward one that recognized the role of risk factors, particularly personal health risk behaviors, and the responsibility of the individual in preventing illness.

The need to address risk factors and lifestyle at the level of public policy found expression in 1974 with the publication in Canada of the *Lalonde Report*. Determinants of health were recognized to include an interaction among factors involving lifestyle, human biology, environment, and health care organization (Lalonde, 1974). By the time *Healthy People: The Surgeon General's Report on Health Promotion and Disease Prevention* (U.S. Department of Health, Education, and Welfare, 1979) appeared in 1979, much had been written about the risk factors for chronic disease. *Healthy People* made recommendations for improved health by summarizing for the American people the connection between personal behavior and health. *Healthy People* was followed in 1980 by *Promoting Health/Preventing Disease: Objectives for the Nation* (U.S. Department of Health and Human Services, 1980), and in 1990 by *Healthy People 2000: National Health Promotion and Disease Prevention Objectives* (U.S. Department of Health and Human Services, 1990), which provided specific objectives for the original priority areas identified in *Healthy People*. The *Healthy People 2000* objectives are organized into three categories: health protection, health promotion, and preventive services. The original 15 priority areas have been expanded to 22 and there are 319 specific objectives to be addressed by the year 2000. Table 8.1 lists the priority areas and provides examples of objectives. *Healthy People 2010* is scheduled for release in 2000.

These federal standards for improving the health of the nation have had a huge impact on organizing institutional public health efforts in the United States. Most public health departments have adopted the

TABLE 8.1   *Healthy People 2000* **Priority Areas and Sample Objectives**

Health promotion
  1. Physical activity and fitness
  2. Nutrition
  3. Tobacco
  4. Alcohol and other drugs
  5. Family planning
  6. Mental health
  7. Violent and abusive behavior
  8. Educational and community-based programs

Health protection
  9. Unintentional injuries
  10. Occupational safety and health
  11. Environmental health
  12. Food and drug safety
  13. Oral health

Preventive services
  14. Maternal and infant health
  15. Heart disease and stroke
  16. Cancer
  17. Diabetes and chronic disabling conditions
  18. HIV infections
  19. Sexually transmitted diseases
  20. Immunization and infectious diseases
  21. Clinical preventive services
  22. Surveillance and data systems

Sample objectives
  1. By 2000, reduce coronary heart disease deaths to no more than 100 per 100,000 people.
  2. By 2000, increase complex carbohydrate and fiber containing food in the diet of adults to 5 or more daily servings for vegetables and fruit, and to 6 or more for grain products.

  3. By 2000, reduce deaths from work-related injuries to no more than 4 per 100,000 full-time workers.

SOURCE: U.S. Department of Health and Human Services (1990).

objectives as the foundation for program development. Although the national standards have added considerably to the development and acceptance of health promotion, they have been criticized for their heavy emphasis on individual behavior. There are also questions about how much effect national centralized planning efforts can really have on the health of people.

Because of the impact of *Healthy People 2000*, and encouraged by the continuing evidence of the role of risk factors in illness, from the latter 1970s on, health program planners have placed considerable emphasis on an individual's ability to choose a healthy lifestyle and

TABLE 8.2   Ottawa Charter for Health Promotion: Prerequisites and Strategies

---

Prerequisites for health
   Peace, shelter, education, food, income, a stable ecosystem, sustainable resources, social justice, and equity
Strategies for action
   Build healthy public policy in all sectors and at all levels
   Create supportive environments
   Strengthen community action, drawing on existing human and material resources to enhance self-help and social support
   Develop personal skills to exercise control over one's own life, health, and environment
   Reorient health services beyond clinical and curative services to focus on total needs of the individual as a whole person

---

SOURCE: World Health Organization (1986).

thus reduce the chances of early death from chronic disease. Health promotion became the theme of an era that ushered in large community health promotion projects, designed primarily to influence personal risk factors for disease.

Moving Beyond Behavior Change

The social context of health promotion and disease prevention was often ignored as technology such as mass media provided an opportunity to bring health education to whole communities. These outside solutions to the community's health, however, often resulted in little long-term impact. It became clear that large-scale, seemingly well-designed projects needed to be community grounded and include institutional and environmental interventions in addition to individual behavior change (Green & Kreuter, 1991). To be successful, projects would have to consider broader, ecological approaches and specifically address the socioenvironmental determinants of the behaviors.

In 1986 in the Ottawa Charter for Health Promotion, the World Health Organization (WHO) emphatically broadened the definition of health promotion beyond personal risk factors and resultant threat of disease (see Table 8.2). The definition includes both the individual and the community roles in addressing all determinants of health. "Health promotion is the process of enabling people to increase control over, and to improve, their health" (World Health Organization [WHO], 1986, p. 425).

Policies in Canada emerged to reflect these considerations in Epp's (1986) report, *Achieving Health for All*. The report recognized the role of socioeconomic inequities and social support in health and supported the WHO definition of health promotion. It recommended a social agenda to solve unaddressed problems in health. That agenda called for greater public involvement in creating health through self care, the decisions people make for themselves to be healthy; mutual aid, the community support needed to help people cope; and healthy environments, the creation of conditions that promote health (Epp, 1986).

Green defines health promotion as "the combination of educational and environmental supports for actions and conditions of living conducive to health" (Green & Kreuter, 1991, p. 4). More broadly, health promotion has been defined as "the aggregate of all purposeful activities designed to improve personal and public health through a combination of strategies, including the competent implementation of behavioral change strategies, health education, health protection measures, risk factor detection, health enhancement, and health maintenance" (Joint Committee on Health Education Terminology, 1991, p. 102).

By the 1990s, appreciation of the impact of social inequities on health led to the linkage of health promotion to various rights advocacy groups. The social justice movement (Labonte, 1993) and the concept of empowerment began to be included in health promotion projects. With roots going back to Freire (1970), empowerment is defined as a "social action process that promotes participation of people, organizations, and communities toward the goals of increased individual and community control, political efficacy, improved quality of community life, and social justice" (Wallerstein, 1992, p. 198).

The need for participation of the people had been articulated by the WHO and the United Nations Children's Fund (UNICEF) at a historic meeting in Alma Ata, in the former U.S.S.R., in 1978, to develop global health policies to promote primary care (WHO & UNICEF, 1978). A report by a WHO committee concluded:

Health science and technology have come to a point where their contribution to the further improvement of health standards can make a real impact only if the people themselves become full partners in health protection and promotion. Too often in the past, "modern" health practices have been promoted without giving sufficient thought to their relevance to the social and cultural background of the communities concerned. An effort must be made to enable individuals and communities to play an active role in the planning and delivery of health care. (World Health Organization Expert Committee, 1983)

Public health policy at the federal level in the United States has been slow in adopting policies that incorporate socioenvironmental approaches, concepts of social equity, and local control. The focus of federal funding and support for health continues to target individuals' diseases and health risk behaviors, rather than addressing the environmental or social circumstances that promote those diseases and behaviors.

Health Protection

Health protection is the use of prevention strategies that are external to the individual, created to shield or protect the individual from injury, harmful exposures, and other external risks. Health protection is usually implemented through statute or regulation. The need for health protection measures is often included in comprehensive health promotion plans. Health protection differs from health promotion, which emphasizes the individual's opportunity to take control over the factors that affect health. The need for health protection is most evident where people are unable to take effective control over the safety and quality of the environment, the safety of what they use, or the safety of the systems they depend on. The long history of public sanitation and environmental control of communicable disease is one of health protection. Health protection strategies additionally may target personal behaviors with intent to address personal safety and health, for example, laws requiring use of seat belts and motorcycle helmets and laws that prohibit the sale of cigarettes to minors.

Implementing health protection. Many health protection steps involve enhancements to the environment that are accepted without contention. In highway safety, for example, requirements for lighting, railings, and standardized signs and lane markings are of undisputed benefit. In the workplace, examples are the use of protective shielding around dangerous machinery and appropriate grounding of electrical equipment. Such enhancements are accepted with little controversy as long as they are not perceived as unreasonably costly.

In other situations, however, mandated health protections result in restriction of freedoms or in unwanted costs and lead to controversy. Laws requiring use of seat belts and motorcycle helmets restrict personal choice and autonomy. Required protective clothing in the workplace may be encumbering or constitute an unwelcome expense. In economic systems where enterprises are under pressure to maximize production while minimizing costs, attempts to regulate in the name of environmental protection and the health and safety of others may be resisted or opposed. For example, regulation of effluents and stack emissions restricts what is allowed to be dispersed into the air or water, and may require costly interventions by the manufacturer.

Policies regulating exposure and risk require accurate assessment of risk. Total elimination of hazards from the environment is unattainable. Risk assessment can be a challenge particularly when the exposures are at low levels, with residual uncertainties that allow room for conflicting conclusions. Approaches to develop regulations and standards in the face of uncertainties about risk and conflicting views about whose rights take precedence are influenced by ideological values. Economic considerations inevitably play a role. Actual enactment of enabling statutes and the development and enforcement of standards are dependent on obtaining support and achieving success within the political process.

Programs to carry out health protection are often administered by regulating and enforcement agencies, such as the Occupational Safety and Health Administration (OSHA) and the Environmental Protection Agency (EPA), that are separate from public health. Roles for public health are to conduct the basic epidemiology that identifies the environmental risk factors, to assess the extent of the problem, to monitor outcomes, and to conduct research. A major additional role for public health is to provide the advocacy and mobilization of public awareness and support needed to generate the necessary political response.

Environmental pollution. Everyone shares the air and depends on access to safe water. People also expect that the land on which they live is without important hazardous contamination. Pollutants include chemical toxins and irritants, heavy metals including lead, pesticides, hazardous dusts, infectious agents, and ionizing radiation. Allergens and noise can also be environmental pollutants.

Compared with federal agencies, state and local environmental control agencies should have the advantages of being more proximate to the sources of pollution and more immediately responsive to the people affected. Without consistent policies across jurisdictions, however, and often without adequate funding, state and local departments of environment are limited in what they can achieve, particularly in protecting the overall quality of the air and major sources of water and in handling problems that cross state boundaries. Congressional recognition of the deterioration of the environment in the United States led to the creation of the EPA in 1970. The EPA is the principal agency to administer previously scattered federal programs and take responsibility to regulate and control many of the major sources of environmental pollution.

Special authorization and funding to clean up existing sites of major ground and water contamination, known as the Super Fund, is administered by the Agency for Toxic Substances and Disease Registry (ATSDR) within the Department of Health and Human Services. The Nuclear Regulatory Commission (NRC) regulates and monitors the use and disposal of radioactive materials.

Whether done nationally or locally, enforcing regulations, conducting environmental monitoring, and abatement of problems require the support and involvement of environmental laboratories, environmental engineers, and technicians. These efforts should be linked with careful epidemiological assessment of health impact. Risk assessment and risk communication skills are essential, as is the backing of the political leadership. In emergency situations where there is an immediate, serious threat to the public, public health officials may intervene directly to control the source and reduce public exposure. Thus, an authorized public health official could impound food products suspected to be contaminated from a market's shelves.

Safety and health in the workplace. The workplace can be a particularly hazardous environment, with risks of injury and illness from many sources. An unremitting record of worker deaths and injury, punctuated by disasters, led to passage of the Occupational Safety and Health Act of 1970. This act set forth protections for the right of workers to protest unsafe working conditions and established OSHA within the Department of Labor with authority to make and enforce health and safety standards that apply to most civilian workplaces. Work-related injuries and illnesses must be reported to OSHA. Workers must be allowed access to information about hazardous chemicals used where they work.

Separate statutory authorities exist to provided protections for miners and agricultural workers. The Department of Defense (DOD) has responsibility for environments at military installations and for maintaining worker safety and health.

The National Institute for Occupational Safety and Health (NIOSH), which is within the CDC, conducts basic research on work-related illness and injury, conducts health hazard evaluations, monitors disease and injury, disseminates information, and supports the training of occupational health professionals. NIOSH recommends and promotes health protection strategies, but does not have regulatory authority. Although worker health and safety are public health issues, responsibility for carrying out health protection activities for workers falls to OSHA and other agencies that are largely removed from public health.

Hazards in daily life. Beyond the general environment and the workplace, there are multiple additional areas that present risks for injury, illness, and death to a vulnerable public. Unsafe commercial products, incompletely evaluated pharmaceuticals and medical devices, sale of contaminated food, defective automobiles and other unsafe systems and vehicles for transportation, unsafe housing including exposure to paints containing lead, and misuse of pesticides are examples. Accordingly, health protection legislation has emerged, often creating agencies to regulate these types of problems. At the national level, examples include the Consumer Product Safety Commission, the Food and Drug Administration, and the Federal Aviation Administration. Other agencies within the Departments of Agriculture, Transportation, and Housing and Urban Development also have regulatory responsibilities for various aspects of safety and health protection and provide support for some initiatives administered at the state level.

Health protection measures are developed through policy, legislation, and regulation. Most commonly, they seek to influence the environment to preserve the individual's health and safety in ways in which the individual need not take on an active role. In this way, they are more limited than the full breadth of health promotion, where interventions seek to empower the individual or community to solve its health related problems.

Additional Reading

McLeroy, K. R., Bibeau, D., Steckler, A., & Glanz, K. (1988). An ecological perspective on health promotion program. *Health Education Quarterly, 15*(4), 351-377.

Chapter 9

Personal Health Care Services

As noted in Chapters 2 and 3, public health in the United States has a long history of providing direct, individual health care services, particularly for persons who lack access to the private medical care system. A major concern of public health is that all people have access to basic health care services, including primary care and preventive services. This is expressed directly in the objectives of *Healthy People 2000* (U.S. Department of Health and Human Services, 1990) and *Healthy Communities 2000: Model Standards* (American Public Health Association, 1991).

As noted in Chapter 3, the role of public health as a provider of direct services is presently under review and in the midst of change. Changes in the financing and structure of medical care have resulted in coverage for greater numbers of people. There is no system, however, to ensure universal coverage and the scope of services covered do not always address issues of significance to public health. As public resources are increasingly drawn into the financing of medical care, there is increased competition for the funds that finance public health's core services.

Chapter 8 describes the triad—health promotion, health protection, and preventive services—used in *Healthy People 2000* (U.S. Department of Health and Human Services, 1990) to provide the framework for organizing the health goals and their respective preventive interventions. This chapter describes public health's role in providing personal health care services.[1] Personal health care services are specific clinical services provided to individuals. Examples of personal health care services are services to diagnose and treat illness and preventive checkups and screenings.

The range of direct personal health care services that is provided by public health is broad. Focused preventive services such as an immunization campaign and categorically organized clinical care services for persons with specific contagious disease such as sexually transmitted disease or tuberculosis are familiar roles for public health departments. Public health may offer comprehensive services, including hospitalization for persons with behavioral health conditions or persons with severe disabilities, when such individuals are unable to find services in the private medical system. Public health may take on the full provision of primary care and even basic hospital services for persons living in medically underserved communities.

The personal health care services discussed in this chapter include clinical preventive services, specifically categorically organized service programs, and full acute and chronic clinical care services. Also covered in this chapter are some of the areas that have implications for health care policy including the relationship between public health and the medical care delivery system, with specific reference to managed care, and the role of cost-effectiveness analysis in resource allocation.

Clinical Preventive Services

One way of categorizing clinical preventive services is to sort by whether an activity is primary, secondary, or tertiary. These terms operate within the disease model, in which a person either is at risk for having or actually has a disease. Primary, secondary, and tertiary prevention apply to persons who are without disease (but at risk), with presymptomatic (occult) disease, and with known disease respectively .

Primary prevention. Primary prevention is the prevention of disease or reduction of risk for disease in the nondiseased person. Immunization is one example of primary prevention, reducing the risk of clinically important infection. Chemoprophylaxis, taking medication to prevent disease, is also primary prevention. Examples of chemoprophylaxis include the use of postmenopausal estrogen to prevent osteoporosis and heart disease in women, the use of aspirin to prevent heart attacks, and the use of mefloquin to prevent malaria in travelers. Counseling to prevent risky behaviors such as tobacco use or to promote healthy diets, exercise, and seat belt use is another example of primary prevention.

Primary prevention strategies operate by reducing the person's risk, either by reducing host susceptibility or by reducing exposure to potentially harmful agents or situations. Looked at broadly, primary prevention can be seen to extend beyond personal health care services to include general health promotion and health protection. The practice of primary prevention at the population level is well known in public health. Fluoridation of public water supplies to reduce incidence of dental caries is an example.

Secondary prevention. Secondary prevention is the identification and early treatment of disease. Secondary prevention is accomplished through screening of persons for previously unknown and usually asymptomatic disease. Examples from cancer prevention are the Pap test to screen for cancer of the cervix, the mammogram to screen for breast cancer, and fecal occult blood testing to screen for colorectal cancer. Other examples are screening newborns for phenylketonuria, thyroid disease, and sickle cell disease; screening children for toxic levels of lead; and screening workers at risk for acoustic injury for hearing loss. For secondary prevention to make sense, the condition being sought should benefit from early detection and intervention. For example, studies have documented that early identification and treatment of cancers of the cervix, breast, and colon improve survival rates. This is not true for all cancers. After controlled trials failed to demonstrate benefit in terms of its reducing mortality from lung cancer, use of chest x-rays and sputum cytology to screen asymptomatic smokers for early lung cancer is no longer recommended (U.S. Preventive Task Force, 1986, chap 11).

The yield from screening increases when the persons selected for screening are known to be at relatively greater risk, based perhaps on age, race, or risk exposure. This increases program efficiency and improves use of limited resources. (See Chapter 5 for a discussion of sensitivity, specificity, and predictive value of screening tests.)

Tertiary prevention. Tertiary prevention takes place in the situation where a person is known to have the disease. It is directed at slowing disease progression, reducing risks of recurrences or complications, and prolonging life. Although one might stretch this definition to include virtually any aspect of medical treatment, it is intended to include such clinical activities as foot care to reduce amputations in diabetics, use of beta-blocking agents to reduce rates of recurrence in patients recovering from heart attacks, and use of aspirin to reduce rates of recurrent strokes. Tertiary prevention shares with secondary prevention the fact that the target subjects have disease. It is distinct from both primary and secondary prevention in that primary and secondary prevention apply strategies widely across populations of asymptomatic individuals, whereas tertiary prevention targets individual patients.

Not every individually targeted preventive step falls neatly within this schema. For example, screening for hypertension and for hypercholesterolemia, both risk factors for coronary artery disease and cerebrovascular disease, may be regarded as primary prevention with respect to heart attack and stroke. At the same time, both hypertension and hypercholesterolemia are themselves regarded as disease conditions, not simply as risk factors. Accordingly, the screening might be viewed as secondary prevention using the above definition. Although one needs to be aware of such ambiguities in the definitions, it does not serve any useful purpose to argue over them. It is important to recognize that hypertension and hypercholesterolemia are important risk conditions, which, if left untreated, will raise the probability of serious vascular disease.

Cost-effectiveness. "An ounce of prevention is worth a pound of cure." Interestingly, the truth is that this is often not the case. Not all prevention activities eventually save money. The dollar cost of prevention may greatly exceed the cost of treating the disease that is being prevented (Russell, 1986). The reason for this is that services for primary and secondary prevention are usually spread across entire populations. The aggregate cost may be very large, even when the cost per person for the preventive service appears to be small. For primary prevention, if the incidence of disease is low, the savings from prevented cases may be only a fraction of the aggregate cost of the preventive service. For secondary prevention, if the prevalence of the disease being screened is low, or if the effectiveness of treatment is poor, the cost needed to prevent a single death or avert disability can be high.

The cost of preventing a death from CHD through populationwide screening for high cholesterol and treating those who are detected with cholesterol-lowering drugs is measured in hundreds of thousands of dollars (Tengs et al., 1995). It is arguable, however, that prevention, even if costly, is worth doing. There are, of course, benefits in addition to the life saved. For CHD, there are the reductions of disease incidence and of disability. Targeting persons or subpopulations thought to be at distinctly high risk improves the use of resources.

Even more dramatic can be the costs involved in eliminating low-level environmental contamination, which, in reality, may pose low *absolute risk* for death. Controls for benzene emissions or elimination of sources of asbestos in low-risk situations may cost tens and hundreds of million of dollars per life saved (Tengs et al., 1995). Many preventive measures do produce more savings than costs, however, such as childhood immunizations, tertiary preventive services targeted to prevent recurrence in a survivor of heart attack, and removal of lead from gasoline and from home paint. Cost-effective preventive measures are enhanced when the risk of adverse outcome is high in the targeted group, when there is an effective intervention, and when the per capita cost of delivering the intervention is low.

Cost-effectiveness analysis is a technique used to identify the costs incurred to achieve an outcome. One frequently used outcome measure, years of life saved, focuses on reducing mortality. Another measure, quality-adjusted years of life saved, incorporates morbidity and disability as well as mortality. Public health program planning may use such measures to compare costs and select the strategies that are the most cost-effective.

Cost-effectiveness analysis is very difficult to perform, requiring accurate information about incidence rates, outcomes, rates of error in diagnosis, and direct and indirect costs projected out over long periods of time. Accurate information applicable to the population under consideration may not be available.

Making clinical preventive services available. Clinical preventive services are delivered in many different ways. Tertiary preventive services are patient-specific and are generally used only in the setting of medical follow-up treatment. Primary and secondary preventive services should be incorporated routinely as components of primary medical care. Unfortunately, this does not always happen. Compliance rates for recommended preventive services performed within medical care settings are often low. To address this, preventive services may be specified as reimbursable, or even as a required condition within federally financed medical care. For example, providers of services for infants and children financed through Medicaid must offer routine, scheduled screening as required by the federally mandated Early Periodic Screening, Diagnosis, and Treatment (EPSDT) program.

There are many authoritative sources such as professional groups and governmental advisory panels that set forth guidelines or recommendations for clinical preventive services. These can be very helpful to providers of care. Specific recommendations from different sources, however, sometimes differ. For example, there are differences with respect to the age when routine mammography should be started or when prostate-specific antigen (PSA) should be used to screen for cancer of the prostate. The differences among the guidelines may have large implications relating to the economics and potential benefits of screening. The recommendations of the U.S. Preventive Services Task Force (1996) and the Canadian Task Force on the Periodic Health Examination (1979) are based on careful review of the scientific literature documenting effectiveness with respect to outcomes. These sources have become widely accepted and used as evidence-based guidelines for clinical primary and secondary prevention of asymptomatic persons in the clinical setting. Such recommendations are increasingly being incorporated into clinical practice guidelines.

Categorical Programs

Organized public health often provides personal preventive and treatment services by way of categorical grant programs (see Chapter 2), which focus on a single disease or clinical issue. *Categorical programs* may emphasize primary preventive services, for example, immunization, or target special populations such as persons with AIDS. Categorical programs in maternal and child health use primary and secondary prevention. Prenatal nutritional counseling is an example of primary prevention, and screening and referring mothers and their infants for high-risk conditions is secondary prevention. Family planning programs include counseling and clinical services. Programs for tuberculosis (TB), for sexually transmitted diseases (STDs), and for HIV/AIDS combine screening, treatment, and education. Other separate programs emphasize a combination of public education and screening, such as cancer, hypertension, diabetes, lead poisoning, and sickle cell disease control programs. Some programs deal with health risk behaviors such as tobacco, drug, and alcohol use, emphasizing education, and may or may not offer individual intervention such as screening, referral, or counseling.

Categorical public health programs offering direct personal services have emerged for several reasons. For communicable diseases such as STDs and TB, case identification, treatment, and follow-up and identification and screening of contacts are essential elements for communitywide control. The private medical system is not oriented or structured for these functions. Special skills, follow-up techniques, and laboratory support are needed for successful intervention in disease rate reduction.

In addition, the development of these and other programs has been encouraged by the availability of categorical funding under either federal or state statute. Such funding may be channeled by way of grants-in-aid to health departments through programs of the Centers for Disease Control and Prevention (CDC) and the National Institutes of Health (NIH). Foundations and nongovernmental organizations that raise their own funding have financed and encouraged categorically specific programs. Examples are plentiful and include heart disease, lung disease, diabetes, birth defects, sickle cell disease, and many others. Advocacy groups have played a major role in lobbying for legislation that mandates categorical programs.

Categorical programs that address individual diseases proceed on the assumption that prevention through counseling, screening, and early intervention will achieve significant reductions of morbidity and mortality. In many instances such programs have been successful in reaching persons who otherwise would be without effective preventive care and treatment. Categorical programs may target such populations with free or low-cost services. Immunization programs, combined with policies requiring immunization before starting school, have contributed to improved overall rates of immunization and marked reductions in incidence of certain infectious disease. The *Women, Infants, and Children (WIC)* nutrition program targets low-income families and accounts for improvements in birth outcomes and in the health of mothers and infants (Rush et al., 1988). Tuberculosis control programs also have been effective.[2]

A limitation of categorical programs is the specificity of their focus. Fragmentation of services often requires an individual to find multiple points of entry to meet different needs. Integration of programs and services may be inadequate or lacking altogether. The specificity of focus also diverts attention away from addressing the social and environmental determinants that have a general effect on health.

In addition, when the public health agenda is driven by categorically restricted funding, opportunity for local determination of priorities and allocation of resources may be preempted. Plans to redirect federal funds for states' programs into general block grants called performance partnership grants and away from categorically restricted grants-in-aid address this issue. States would determine the priorities, and accountability under these block grants would be in the state's demonstration that specific health outcome goals have been reached. Block grants may also be used as a means of cutting back overall levels of federal support.

Primary Care and General Medical Services

Primary care and general medical services include care of persons who may be ill with anything, not necessarily conditions of particular public health significance such as those addressed by categorical programs. When ordinary medical care services are not accessible, public health may be called to step in. Access to needed health care services is a core assurance function of public health. Governmentally sponsored health care activities take many forms. Government may provide the financing for private health care, or may directly operate primary care clinics. Federally qualified health centers (FQHCs) are publicly subsidized primary care clinics in underserved inner-city neighborhoods and rural areas. The governmental financing of clinical services for poor people through Medicaid has removed financial barriers to access to private sector services and encouraged expansion of private health care into previously underserved areas. Funding for facilities and services may flow through state and local or municipal health departments.

In addition, the federal government has several specific health care delivery programs. The National Health Service Corps recruits and places physicians, dentists, and other professional staff in underserved areas. The Indian Health Service has been an integrated system of clinical health care services managed by the U.S. Public Health Service since 1954 when it was transferred from the Bureau of Indian Affairs. The Department of Veterans Affairs manages a system of clinics and hospitals for veterans.

Public Health and the Medical Care Delivery System

Public health encourages the private sector to involve itself with providing clinical preventive services that address public health goals by providing public financing of medical care services. The use of *managed care organizations* (MCOs; see Chapter 3) to provide medical services could increase opportunity for specifying the provision of preventive services.

MCOs provide specific, covered medical services to enrolled patients. In the United States in the 1980s and 1990s with massive capitalization, MCOs have secured an advantage in the competitive health care marketplace, especially in urban areas. MCOs have come to be recognized by purchasers of health care services as more cost effective than the fee-for-service system (see Chapter 3).

When services are provided through MCOs using public funds, such as for persons receiving Medicaid and Medicare, public financing entities have responsibilities to regulate and monitor the delivery and quality of basic preventive services. This is an opportunity for the insertion of a public health perspective. This applies, for example, to a state public health input into the design of Medicaid managed care. Publicly financed contracts should require provisions for immunizations, screening, and other basic clinical preventive services; protection of enrollees' timely access to needed services; consumer input into program planning; open enrollment; choice of primary care provider; and timely handling of grievances. In addition, MCOs must report reportable diseases and cooperate in the control of outbreaks.

Of additional public concern is the unwillingness of some MCOs to enroll and retain people who are at high risk or who have special needs. MCOs, seeking to be financially competitive, may have policies that discourage enrollment. Such policies have a negative public health effect by denying persons with medical needs access to services. Persons identified as possible consumers of a disproportionate share of the health care dollar must not be excluded from the health care system.

Notes

1. The history of provision of personal health services as a direct public responsibility within public health is a long one. In the United States, the Marine Hospital System was established at the end of the 18th century (see Chapter 1). In the first half of the 20th century, public health clinics emerged to broaden use

of immunizations for children in an effort to curb spread of infection. As it became apparent that many children did not have effective access to general preventive care through the regular medical care system, well child clinics were established. Prenatal clinics followed. In the 1960s, with federal grants, full-service, community-based primary care clinics started to appear.

2. Some of the increase in spread of tuberculosis that began in areas of the United States in the 1980s is attributable to the premature complacency that tuberculosis was a receding concern and to the downsizing and elimination of tuberculosis control programs in many departments of health.

Chapter 10

Health Program Planning

―――――――――――――― ᦂᦖ ――――――――――――――

Health planning can take many forms. Over the years there have been many attempts at national, comprehensive health planning, but most have ended in frustration and dissolution. Currently, planning occurs at the state, regional, and local levels, at the agency level and in health care delivery systems. Planning can be viewed as an attempt to make objective decisions to reach a certain desired outcome. For the purpose of this chapter, *health planning* is defined as the orderly process of developing, implementing, and evaluating health programs. Health program planning depends on the analytical tools and epidemiology of public health. Program planning can be very complex, beginning with an analysis of health and social problems and ending with an examination of the effectiveness of the project itself. Planning encompasses needs assessment, setting of priorities, program development, implementation, and evaluation. This chapter provides a brief, general overview for health promotion program planning, expanding on those concepts of health promotion and prevention discussed in earlier chapters. This chapter is intended to provide an overview; it is not intended to thoroughly address the steps in health planning nor the advantages and disadvantages of the methods presented.

The essential concept that will be discussed throughout this chapter is that although program planning depends on quantitative data, it also develops in a social context. Adequately defining problems requires a value judgment, a social decision-making process. Facts can be accumulated, but people give them meaning. A problem for one group may not cause concern for others. Appropriate program planning must include quantitative facts as well as qualitative judgments about the problem.

Public health planning often is a "top down" process, starting with government agencies. Health department planners have access to the health statistics for a community, and are in a position to see what health problem exists. With all good intentions, health planners proceed to develop a community plan and intervention from "outside" the community. Developing plans from the outside, however, can ignore the social context of the problem. Who is experiencing the problem? It is very unlikely that everyone in the community is experiencing the problem equally. Who should be involved in the planning process? How is the community defined?

Even with determination that health planning will be done from within a community, these questions are difficult to answer. Communities are complex, and subgroups have their own concerns and priorities. It is difficult to have balanced representation of all constituencies at the planning table. Public health programs ultimately promote change, and program implementation may not benefit everyone equally. Changes in individual behavior or in collective community action can pose threats to established methods of operation, and efforts toward health could result in harm for some in a population. The methods inherent in a program's intervention strategies can result in consequences that reduce independence and affect economic conditions for individuals. Basic to all health program planning activities should be a thorough examination of the ethical issues that can be problematic in any program that is advocating change.

Basic Principles in Ethics

Classically, four basic principles comprise the foundation of health ethics. They are justice, beneficence, nonmaleficence, and autonomy (Last, 1992).

Justice. Justice deals with equity and the fair distribution of public resources and protection. All people should have fair and equal opportunity for access to the fruits and social benefits derived from the use of public resources; all persons should be protected equally and impartially, without having to incur burdens or risks that might result from others' gain or advantage. The principle of justice underlies public health's responsibility to reduce gaps in health status found between groups and social classes. Distributive justice is the application of resources to meet the needs of the poor and disadvantaged. It addresses the direct relationship between a group's share of the total wealth and its health status.

Beneficence. Beneficence is to do what is for the good or welfare of another. When there are choices, beneficence implies doing the most good for the most people. Beneficence underlies the core functions of policy development and assurance in public health. The overriding goal of public health to improve and assure the health of populations rests on the principle of beneficence.

Nonmaleficence. Nonmaleficence is the avoidance of doing harm. Many public health programs entail risks that accompany the benefits. Polio vaccines illustrate the point. The widespread use of orally administered vaccine containing live attenuated virus has resulted in the elimination of naturally occurring polio in many parts of the world. The live virus, however, carries a small, but very real risk of causing paralytic disease. When natural polio was a large threat, the risk of vaccine-associated complication was accepted. Where natural polio is eradicated, the acceptability is questioned under the principle of nonmaleficence. Accordingly, policymakers have recommended polio immunization schedules that include the use of vaccines made from killed virus, which require injection. These are safer, but more costly and difficult to administer.

Autonomy. Autonomy is the right of a person to make decisions on his or her own behalf. Autonomy values individual dignity, self-worth, intelligence, and capacity for choice. It respects liberty. Informed consent before health care treatment, for example, is meant to protect an individual's autonomy. Antismoking campaigns can be seen as violating the rights of smokers. Ending tobacco subsidies could put many people out of work. Establishments that serve the public could lose clientele because of smoking regulations. Weighing the beneficial and harmful effects is important to health program planning.

Each of these principles should command the attention and respect of anyone having responsibility for actions that affect others. Indeed, one should challenge any action that cannot be justified in terms of at least one of these principles. Ethical dilemmas arise when an action advanced under one principle runs counter to another. There is hardly an issue in public health that does not have to confront ethical dilemmas at some level. Conflicts among the ethical principles cannot always be fully resolved, but analysis of any situation using the principles can be of great value in untangling and understanding differences in viewpoints. Moral values, religious views, and political environments may be helpful in clarifying the ethical principles. They should not be used to silence discourse or to rigidly dictate how differences are reconciled.

The following are examples of conflicts faced in the course of carrying out public health activities. To protect the public from the spread of communicable disease, contagious or potentially infectious individuals must be identified and isolated. This presents an obvious conflict between beneficence and autonomy, and should be undertaken only when risks to the public are serious and credible. Similarly, to eradicate a point source of infection such as a food supplier, the necessary steps may infringe on individual or corporate freedoms or economic interests. To protect the public from the effects of environmental pollution, steps must be taken to curb individual and corporate polluters. Just as with those responsible for point source infections, regulation may infringe on individual or corporate autonomy and may generate short-run costs. This is of particular concern in a competitive market economy in which production efficiencies are necessary for economic survival. Adding expensive clean-up equipment, for example, may be so costly as to make the product less competitive.

Theory and Models for Individual Change

Theories and models form the basis for health program planning and evaluation. Theories are principles and propositions that explain a situation or event. They are abstract and broad in their application; they attempt to organize and explain the underlying processes that account for an observable event. Theory helps explain what influences health-related behavior. According to van Ryn and Heaney (1992), theories can provide answers as to why people are not engaging in healthy behaviors, how to go about changing those behaviors, and what factors to look for in evaluating program effectiveness. Theories explain, but no one theory provides the perfect explanation. Therefore, no one theory predominates in health education and research. Theories can be thought of as conceptual frameworks to provide guidelines in the planning process, and disease prevention programs often have more than one theory as a basis for intervention. *Models* are plans, generalized descriptions that are also used to explain events. Models do not attempt to explain the underlying theoretical principles in the social and behavioral sciences, for example, but do incorporate theory into their design. They are the application of theory.

Because of the increased emphasis over the years on individual behavior change in health promotion, health planners have given considerable attention to theories that shed light on why individuals do what they do. These theories are usually cognitive-behavioral in nature. Concepts inherent in these theories are that behaviors are mediated through what one knows and thinks, but knowledge alone does not produce change. There are other factors influencing behavior besides those that are internal to the individual. People exist in a social environment where the thoughts and advice of others affect their own behavior.

Social learning theory. Social learning theory is a cognitive-behavioral theory that assumes a constant interaction between individuals and their environment. Behavior is influenced by internal factors and modified by external factors. Social learning, or social cognitive theory, proposed by Bandura (1986) is a commonly used theory in health

promotion. Basic to this model is the concept of reciprocal deter-
minism, that behavior changes result from interpersonal and environmental interactions. Individuals are constantly changing their environment and being changed by that environment. Change is
reciprocal and continual (Bandura, 1986). To change health behavior
an individual must also have the behavioral capability or knowledge
and skills to know what to do. The individual's self-efficacy to take
action is highly important as is the observational learning that takes
place as others are observed in their behaviors. People model their
behavior and the consequences for others to examine. Famous, powerful, or highly respected people can often influence others. They are
commonly used in health promotion activities as promoters of behavior change. Reinforcement, such as rewards and praise, increases
the chances that the behavior will recur.

The theory of reasoned action (TRA). This theory, developed by
Fishbein and Ajzen in 1975, presents the four constructs of belief,
attitude, behavioral intention, and behavior as separate and interre-
lated. Basically, behavior is preceded by an intent to engage in the
behavior. The intent is influenced by the person's beliefs and the
attitude toward the behavior, as well as the social environment, or
subjective norm. Relevant others can significantly influence an individual's behavior. To adjust the model to apply to behaviors that are
not completely under an individual's control, Ajzen (1988) extended
the TRA model to the *theory of planned behavior (TPB)*. The TPB adds
another dimension, that of perceived control, to the theory. If a person
is serious about adopting a low-fat diet, he must perceive that he has
control over his eating habits and can succeed. These three theories
are widely applied in health education and health promotion.

Models help in identifying what might be affecting behavior. Three
of the most commonly used frameworks for describing health behavior
are (a) the stages of change model, (b) the health belief model, and (c)
the consumer information processing model.

The stages of change model. Introduced by Prochaska and DiClemente
in 1983, this model views behavior change as a circular process, not
an event. Individuals are at varying degrees of readiness to change and
each stage of readiness can benefit from a different intervention. For

example, smokers might be unaware of a problem and not thinking about changing smoking behavior (precontemplation). Later, the smoker may begin to question the advisability of smoking and begin to think about change (contemplation). At a later time a decision to quit may result in a plan for action (decision/determination). Implementation of the plan (action) and the continuation of the new behavior (maintenance) are phases through which individuals may move in and out. Thus, individuals are in varying stages of change, entering and exiting at any point (National Cancer Institute, 1995).

The health belief model. Formulated by Hochbaum, Rosenstock, Leventhal, and Kegeles for the Public Health Service, the health belief model is one of the most commonly used models in health promotion. The concepts of this model account for an individual's readiness to take a health action. One's belief that he or she could get a disease or condition (perceived susceptibility) and that the condition could be serious (perceived severity) leads to thinking about a health action (perceived benefits). The perceived barriers are then weighed, and the costs versus the benefits of action are assessed. Cues to action, such as the availability of how-to information and the self-efficacy of the individual, also affect the outcome (Rosenstock, Strecher, & Becker, 1988).

The consumer information processing model. This model recognizes that individuals have a limited or finite capacity for processing information. People will use health information if it is useful and easy to process. Applications for health educators are that information prepared for the consumer should be useful, attractive, and take little effort to obtain and integrate (Bettman, 1979).

Theory and Models for Community Change

Several theories and models for community health-related change are commonly used in health program planning, including three stages of community organization for health that have been described by Rothman and Tropman (1987). These are helpful for planning public health activities, because they depict different levels of community involvement and provide a framework for understanding. They are the following: (a) social planning, (b) locality development, and (c) social action.

Social planning. Social planning is task focused, addressing problem solving by using experts from the outside to provide considerable technical support. It continues to be the predominant model in community health planning. Categorical programs, described earlier, generally fall within this model. The plan is developed by "experts," often with little or no community involvement. The agenda and the principal methods are usually set in advance from outside. Generally, such programs need to invest in building awareness and in mobilizing community participation. Unfortunately, employment of this model without community support often fails to achieve outcome objectives.

Locality development. In contrast to social planning, locality development or community development refers to a broad-based representative group of people who identify and solve their own problems. Capacity building and consensus are essential. Often outside advisers are asked for technical assistance, but members of the community are in control of the planning agenda.

Health planning tools developed for communities in the 1980s often provided guidelines for a community process for identifying health problems. One attempt to put the objectives of *Healthy People 2000* into practice in the community is the American Public Health Association's (1991) *Healthy Communities 2000: Model Standards, Guidelines for Community Attainment of the Year 2000 National Health Objectives.* The work encourages communities to establish achievable health targets by adapting the national objectives into locally feasible plans of action.

Other community organization tools have been developed to assist with local health planning. One of these is the *Planned Approach to Community Health,* known by the acronym PATCH, developed by the Centers for Disease Control and Prevention (CDC) in the mid-1980s. The goal of PATCH is to increase the capacity of communities to collect local data, plan, implement, and evaluate comprehensive, community-based health promotion programs targeted toward priority health problems. The CDC promotes the use of PATCH in achieving the *Healthy People 2000* national health objectives. It is organized within the context of the PRECEDE model (Centers for Disease Control and Prevention, 1995b).

Although both of these planning tools can be useful examples of locality development, using the guidelines developed by the CDC and others can also be a disadvantage. Adherence to the guidelines reduces the flexibility of communities to develop their own approach. Ideally, locality development should reach consensus through a broad representation of community members. When this is achieved, locality development has resulted in successful health projects.

Paulo Freire, a Brazilian educator, in his theory of freeing, saw education as the key for empowerment, the power to act with others to effect change. People living in communities become more critically conscious of the problems and develop their own action plans to address them (Freire, 1970).

Projects may start as examples of social planning and evolve into locality/community development as illustrated by the Tenderloin Senior Outreach Organizing Project in San Francisco (Minkler, 1995). This project sought to address the health needs of poor, socially isolated, elderly people living in single-room occupancy hotels. It started with an attempt to use public health students and faculty to improve the residents' physical and mental health by reducing social isolation and offering health education. In addition, participants facilitated a process through which residents were encouraged to identify and seek solutions to common problems. The project gained acceptance and widespread participation only after the residents were able to build trust and rapport, share mutual concerns, and structure program priorities such as issues of safety on the streets. The methods used here drew on the social empowerment theories of Freire (1970).

The growing use of community health workers (CHWs) to act as links between health and human services and people in need is another example of locality development. Although widely used in developing countries, the CHW model is only recently receiving widespread attention in the United States. CHWs are local, indigenous (and usually) women sharing the cultural and ethnic characteristics of their neighbors. They are being used to reach out to provide support and basic health education to those least likely to access services. Evaluations of community health worker programs have shown them to be effective in facilitating access to health care. CHWs can also be instrumental in building community strengths to solve problems (Witmer, Seifer, Finnocchio, Leslie, & O'Neil, 1995).

The Healthy Cities project, sponsored by WHO, attempts to take localities development to a large scale. Originating in Europe, the healthy cities model is now present in several states in the United States and in Canada. The approach ultimately attempts to achieve a social environment that will be effective in solving problems and providing support for its citizens. Inherent in the healthy city's model is a process of community strengthening and empowerment. The city is healthy to the extent that it is able to manage its own problems and expand its resources to support its people. As the management of problems becomes easier and a more just society results, social indicators including the health of the population improve. Changes in health policy and the social environment that support healthier people are basic to the model, which uses locally determined priorities, develops plans, and proceeds by integrating inputs from different municipal agencies and others (Duhl, 1993; Tsouros, 1995).

Social action. Social action is organized community demand for change to address social inequities. When the needs of the people are not being served by the usual kinds of planning for change, often communities choose to take stronger action. Oppressed groups of people band together to achieve social justice. Significant improvement in the health and safety of workers, for example, occurred as a result of the labor movement and the confrontation of management by unions, just as rallies and marches of thousands of people have helped draw attention to AIDS and other important health problems.

Diffusion of innovations theory. It is very useful to understand how new ideas and technology get adopted by the community. Why does the school system select a new curriculum or the organization initiate work site wellness activities? Why do health consumers begin to use one new medical device and not another? Diffusion of innovations theory provides answers to why some ideas and new products are quickly accepted by people and others are not. Concepts within the theory include the following: relative advantage, compatibility, complexity, trialability, and observability. Innovations that offer a relative advantage to the user so that they are seen to be better than the old way are more quickly adopted. Products or ideas that are compatible with the values and habits of users and not too difficult to use or understand are perceived as better. Trialability, or the extent to which the product can be experimented with, seems to affect adoption as does observability, the extent to which the product can provide tangible results. Health projects that include the diffusion of ideas or products are more successful if knowledge of the community's formal and informal communication channels exists (National Cancer Institute, 1995).

Social marketing. Social marketing builds on social learning theory and diffusion of information by adding the techniques used in advertising to influence behavior. This planning tool gained wide acceptance in the 1980s when it was used in several major community cardiovascular risk factor intervention trials. The technique encourages the use of multiple channels of communication, including media, community organizations, and businesses to convey health education messages. The intent is to modify the behavior of individuals toward a healthier lifestyle (Lefebvre & Flora, 1988).

Media advocacy. Media advocacy is the deliberate creation of media events to build support for health policy. It makes use of selective epidemiological information to dramatize the situation (Wallack et al., 1993).

Successful public health campaigns will likely combine more than one theory, model, and intervention technique. Comprehensive community projects will include individual behavior change interventions as well as promote organizational change and policy development.

A Health Planning Model

Appropriate health planning forms the framework for health promotion programs. In general, the steps in health planning are the following: (a) assessing the need; (b) identifying the problem; (c) setting priorities and developing goals and objectives; (d) designing the intervention strategy; (e) implementing the intervention; and (f) evaluating the program.

One widely accepted model in health promotion planning today is the PRECEDE/PROCEED model developed by Green and Kreuter (1991). Advantages of the model include a strong emphasis on the social context of health planning. Social diagnosis in this model promotes self analysis to determine need by the people in the community. In addition to individual behavioral contributors, the steps of the model increasingly recognize and affect the environmental conditions that are contributing to the problem. It is a comprehensive planning model that has been adopted on a national and international scale (see Figure 10.1).

The importance of adequate social diagnosis from within the community is Phase One of the planning process. Green and Kreuter (1991) define social diagnosis as

> the process of determining people's perceptions of their own needs or quality of life, and their aspirations for the common good, through broad participation and the application of multiple information-gathering activities designed to expand understanding of the community. . . . Community participation (broad participation if the client system is other than a geographic community) is a foundation concept in social diagnosis and has long been a basic principle for health education and community development, although too often neglected in practice.
>
> One of the goals of health promotion programs is healthful living patterns and conditions that last. The behavioral and environmental changes induced by the program should have staying power. Programs conceived and developed apart from the spirit and day to day workings of a community are, by definition, outside that community. In such cases, when the initial resources dry up or the intervention period comes to an end, the program is not only over, it is gone! A program that never becomes a real part of the community generates no sense of community ownership and so has little or no chance of becoming a permanent part of the community fabric. To obtain a lasting effect, to achieve a positive shift in a community's health norms, genuine community participation and commitment are essential.

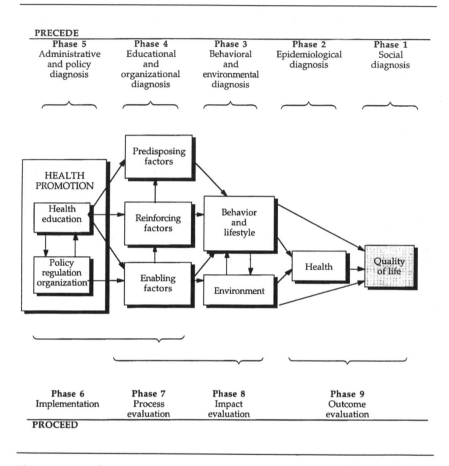

Figure 10.1. The PRECEDE/PROCEED Model

SOURCE: *Health Promotion Planning: An Educational and Environmental Approach*, by Lawrence W. Green and Marshall W. Kreuter. Copyright © 1991 by Mayfield Publishing. Reprinted with permission of the publisher.

The concerns that are identified in Phase 1, the social diagnosis, are supplemented in Phase 2, the epidemiological diagnosis. Specific health problems that may be contributing to the quality of life are identified at this stage. Phase 3 identifies the behavioral and environmental factors that are contributing to the health problems. Phase 4 categorizes those environmental and behavioral contributors into predisposing, enabling, and reinforcing factors. Phase 5 is the administrative assessment of the resources and capabilities to undertake the program. The PROCEED part of the model makes up the implementation and evaluation Phases 6, 7, 8, and 9.

A community with high rates of alcohol abuse, for example, may be experiencing quality-of-life indicators such as increased levels of unemployment, school dropout rates, DWI arrests, motor vehicle fatalities, and domestic violence among others. The epidemiological diagnosis, Phase 2, might confirm the health-related data such as high rates of alcohol-related morbidity and mortality and hospitalized victims of accidents and domestic abuse. This phase would examine the health problems associated with the social problems in Phase 1. Phase 3 would assess the environmental and behavioral factors that are contributing to Phase 1 and 2. Risk factors for alcohol abuse might include poor coping skills or alcohol consumption patterns. Environmental factors such as the availability of alcohol and permissive regulations that encourage its use affect the problem. Phase 4 identifies the predisposing factors, those characteristics of an individual such as knowledge, attitudes, and beliefs that influence behavior. Also in this phase, the enabling and reinforcing factors that influence the problem, such as the availability of community resources and the role of the family, among others, are identified. The administrative and policy diagnosis, Phase 5, would determine how the problem can be addressed. The remaining phases focus on the full development and implementation of the intervention and program evaluation.

Needs Assessment

Every planning process must have an estimate of need. The concept of need can be complex. It is generally assumed to be, at least in public health, the gap between what is desirable and what is actually occurring. Need is relative to existing conditions, not an absolute standard. Need develops in a sociopolitical environment and has objective and subjective components.

A needs assessment is a systematic method of gathering information for the planning process. It can determine the existence of a problem quantitatively by providing numerical support, and qualitatively through opinions that judge or label the facts. Gathering health data for an individual or a population can be done in a variety of ways. During the process, the health planner must be constantly aware of who has the need. What is the purpose of the information gathering? Has the community seen a problem it wants corrected, or has the health planner seen a problem as a result of reviewing recent health statistics? Both are common ways of expressing need. No single source of data provides the complete needs picture. Need is multidimensional, occasionally reported as an absolute standard in health related concerns, but more often viewed to be relative to current conditions. Need is often thought of as not having access to essential goods or services.

Perceived needs are those reported by the people in the community, what they feel their needs are. Perhaps a health planner has been contacted by a community, for example, to assess the need for primary care services. This type of need would be a perceived need if most community members felt (qualitative) there was not enough access to primary care services. A survey (quantitative) of primary care providers in the area, however, might indicate that there were enough practicing to meet the federal standard of 1 per 1,500 population, thus meeting the normative need. At this point it might seem as if there were no real need. If, however, those providers were in private practice and were refusing to see uninsured or Medicaid patients, then there could be a real need for more providers to treat these groups. Or perhaps an unusually high percentage of people work during the daytime in this community, so that there is a need for after hours and weekend care, which may not be currently provided. The relative nature of need is thus affected by circumstances including demographics, which strongly influence what people need.

Health information gathered from public health monitoring and surveillance systems provide epidemiological data, which often form the basis for health planning. Community members may not agree with the priorities that may be derived from the health statistics that define their problems, however. High rates of heart disease may not concern a community as much as violence, for example. It is the job of a health planner to obtain an accurate picture of need by blending health statistics and community concerns, ideally producing a project that will serve the needs of the people.

The three most commonly used methods of assessing the subjective needs and concerns of groups of people are the focus group, the nominal group process, and the Delphi technique. These techniques can provide essential qualitative information for diagnosing problems.

Focus group. The focus group is commonly used to bring community members together in an informal setting to provide opinions about a specific issue. This technique is useful in all stages of planning. Although groups need to remain small (not more than 15 people), several focus groups on the same issue can elicit the opinions of a variety of community representatives. Thus, the focus group is a relatively informal meeting that brings together somewhat homogeneous groups of people. A skilled facilitator is necessary to guide the group through the process. The focus group can be an inexpensive method to assess community beliefs. Usually a single question is posed to each focus group. It could be broadly stated, such as a question about the major health concerns in the community, or have a more narrow focus, such as defining specific objectives in a health plan.

Nominal group process. The nominal group process is an excellent way of identifying and ranking problems. The process can quickly produce a number one priority from a group, and, like the Delphi technique, has the advantage of giving participants an equal voice, preventing any one person from controlling the outcome. The process brings together a few knowledgeable people to write responses to a specific question without discussion among themselves. Each participant then shares his or her response to the question and these responses are then prioritized in importance by the group. The final step includes a numerical ranking that quantifies the results of the process.

Delphi technique. The Delphi technique is a method of reaching group consensus to a specific question through the use of a mailed questionnaire. Usually 10 to 15 knowledgeable people are asked to respond. Because the Delphi technique can be conducted by mail, it has the advantage of including geographically separated individuals, if necessary. Through the process of ranking the results of the question-naires a consensus is reached. The steps to conducting a Delphi technique are described by Gilmore and Campbell (1996).

Surveys, questionnaires, and interviews are other preferred methods of eliciting individual responses for health planning pur-poses. Surveys by mail, telephone, and face-to-face interviews are commonly used assessment techniques. The information gathered from surveys can be quantitative or qualitative. Once the information from the needs assessment is gathered, the analysis must begin. The problem(s) or the purpose of the program must be identified, and the goals and objectives developed. The purpose of the project can serve as the guiding force for further development. It is generally a very broad statement or two summarizing the program ideals. For example, the XYZ Corporation wants employees to reach their full potential. The corporation will assist employees to become healthier by providing on-site opportunities to participate in physical fitness and smoking cessation activities.

Goals and Objectives

When the purpose of the project is well defined, it is time to formulate the goals and objectives that will achieve the purpose. *Goals* are broad, abstract statements of intent. Goals provide direction. Goals should tell what is going to happen as a result of the project. Goals are general, nonspecific, and easily supported by nearly everyone. Goals such as "improved health for children" can help bring disparate groups together working toward a valued social accomplishment.

Objectives are measurable, specific statements that lead toward the goals and define what change will take place. Action steps are methods and activities to accomplish the objectives. Objectives should answer the following questions: who, what, how much, and when. Objectives need to be clear and well defined. Because they form the foundation for program evaluation, they should be measurable. It is often difficult to ascertain certain conditions such as whether or not program participants understand the information. Therefore, designing objectives that build in a demonstration of understanding is preferable. "Of the participants in the first class, 90% will be able to list the five major risk factors for heart disease as determined by the quiz at the end of the session" instead of "90% will understand the risk factors by the end of the session." Objectives can address long-term outcome as well as short-term program functions. Reduced deaths due to coronary heart disease would be measured over a period of years following the program, whereas the development of a screening instrument would be assigned a more immediate time frame. Both can be measured by well-written objectives. Action steps become the intervention, what is going to be done to achieve the goals and objectives.

An example of a health project goal would be to improve the health status of the residents of Merryville. An objective to support the goal might be the following: Increase the number of women in the community who receive mammograms every 2 years from 20% to 35% by the end of the project period. An action step to support the objective might be to organize a yearly health fair in Merryville, which will provide health education and screening information on breast cancer prevention.

Intervention strategies must be realistic. They must be acceptable to the community. Strategies for intervention are most effective when they include the social, environmental, and policy arenas as well as behavior change.

Evaluation

Program evaluation, or how well the program did what it intended to do, actually occurs at many levels throughout the course of the project and afterward. Evaluation produces information about the success of the project and about those pieces that did not work well. Documenting failure is also part of evaluation, because most projects are not perfectly executed. Often the information gained from what did not work is very helpful. Well-written objectives assist the evaluation process. Evaluation looks at all aspects of a health promotion program including whether or not the long-term outcome was better health as formulated by the program goal. Evaluation standards should be decided before the program starts, and an "action" model of evaluation provides continuous information to assist in program adjustment when needed.

Process evaluation assesses the service and administrative parts of the program. It includes an examination of the effectiveness of the staff, the amount and quality of services provided, interactions with staff and program recipients, the content of the materials, and budget review among other components.

Impact evaluation assesses whether or not change occurred as a result of the program. It usually examines short-term changes—such as, how many people quit smoking as a result of the program. Impact evaluation would determine if the immediate program objectives were met.

Outcome evaluation assesses whether or not the project had a long-term effect. It may demonstrate the effectiveness of the program to reach its goals, such as a reduction in heart disease. Health-related programs often measure changes in health status to judge ultimate program effectiveness. Evaluation also includes cost efficiency and cost-effectiveness information.

Good health planning recognizes that most communities will not have the resources to adequately address all the community health concerns. Health planning includes prioritizing problems as well as assessing the capacity to solve them. Translating data into a meaningful plan for action must include the political will and the community resources to make it happen.

Chapter 11

Global
Health

The health of people living in the world's developed countries has generally improved over the past several decades. The same cannot be said for the vast numbers who live in many countries of the developing world. Table 11.1 lists some of the grim facts pertaining to the widening gaps between the two worlds. Whereas life expectancy is increasing in the most developed countries, it is actually shrinking in some of the poorest. Seen in the contexts of increasing population size, massive urbanization, extreme poverty, environmental degradation, and inadequate international response, the world appears to be heading toward a health catastrophe (World Health Organization [WHO], 1995).

TABLE 11.1 Facts About World Health

- The world's population has more than doubled from 2.5 billion in 1950 to 5.6 billion in 1995, including 4.4 billion in the developing world.
- More than one fifth of the global population lives in extreme poverty.
- Life expectancy in one of the world's least developed countries is 43 years, compared with 78 years in one of the world's most developed countries.
- Despite gains in overall life expectancy—a rise of 4 years to 65 years since 1980—at least 5 countries will see their life expectancy rates drop in the next 5 years.
- Half of the world's population lacks regular access to treatment of common diseases and to the most needed essential drugs.
- Up to 320 out of every 1,000 babies do not reach their 5th birthday in some parts of the developing world, compared with only 6 deaths under 5 years per 1,000 births in some of the most developed countries. In developing countries in 1993, 12.2 million children died from the following:

    4 million deaths from acute respiratory infection

    3 million deaths from diarrhea

    2.4 million from vaccine-preventable disease
- The number of street children is estimated to be 100 million.
- Of all deaths, 40% are caused by communicable disease.
- The largest causes of death are diseases of the heart and circulatory systems, resulting in 10 million deaths per year.
- Overall, the effects of smoking kill 6 people a minute. Smoking is the world's largest single preventable cause of illness and death. It already kills 3 million people a year and is expected to kill 10 million by the year 2020.

SOURCE: Adapted from World Health Organization (1995).

Determinants of Health in a Changing World

Beneath the diseases are the situations and underlying conditions that constitute immediate determinants (Table 11.2). At an even more fundamental level, asserts the World Health Organization (WHO), is poverty, especially extreme poverty:

> Poverty is the main reason why babies are not vaccinated, why clean water and sanitation are not provided, why curative drugs and other treatments are unavailable, and why mothers die in childbirth. It is the underlying cause of reduced life expectancy, handicap, disability, and starvation. Poverty is a major contributor to mental illness, stress, suicide, family disintegration, and substance abuse. Every year in the developing world, 12.2 million children under 5 years die, most of

TABLE 11.2 Estimated Number and Percentage of Deaths Worldwide Attributed to Ten Major Risk Factors in 1990

	Deaths	
Risk Factor	Estimated Number	Percentage of Total Deaths
Malnutrition	5,881,000	11.7
Tobacco use	3.038,000	6.0
Hypertension	2,918,000	5.8
Poor water supply, sanitation, and hygiene	2,668,000	5.3
Physical inactivity	1,991,000	3.9
Occupation	1,129,000	2.2
Unsafe sex	1,095,000	2.2
Alcohol	774,000	1.5
Air pollution	568,000	1.1
Illicit drug use	100,000	0.2

SOURCE: Murray and Lopez (1996, Table 3).

them from causes that could be prevented for just a few U.S. cents per child. They die largely because of world indifference, but most of all they die because they are poor. (WHO, 1995)

The gaps between the developed and developing world continue to widen. The dominant international economic system is characterized by enormous concentrations of corporate wealth and access to investment capital, opportunities and incentives that reduce tax obligations, policies that promote open trading and flow of capital and access to unprotected labor markets. The system allows ready access to natural resources with little restraint on environmental impact. The result can be disproportionate benefit to the groups within nations that are already the most wealthy. The economic system and policies are indifferent to issues of distributive justice, particularly in the absence of international standards to ensure fair labor practices and environmental protections.

Measures of national wealth only roughly correlate with national health indexes such as infant mortality and life expectancy. The correlation is strengthened after adjusting for uneven distribution of wealth within each country (Roemer, 1985, chap. 4). Thus, except at levels of extreme poverty, the specific level of poverty may not be the determining variable. Rather, increased degree of social gradient and lack of equality in the distribution of wealth within a population directly predict reduced life expectancy (Wilkinson, 1992). The phenomenon of the effect of the magnitude of the social gradient on mortality is observable in every country. Even among the most developed countries, the more adverse rates of outcome are seen in association with the wider spreads in social distribution of wealth, suggesting that social inequality is an intrinsic determinant of overall health status (Evans, Barer, & Marmor, 1994). This observation bodes poorly for a world beset with population pressures, joblessness, poverty, and a widening gap between the rich and the poor.

The independent association of poor social support with cardiovascular disease has been documented (Berkman, 1986). The connection between social class and mortality was demonstrated in the Whitehall study in England (Marmot, Kogevinas, & Elston, 1987). A three- to fivefold mortality differential was observed between the extremes of social class. The differential could not be accounted for by distribution of known determinants of risk such as tobacco use.

Level of education plays a vital and consistently observed role in health across all populations. For example, a woman's health is heavily dependent on numbers of children and their spacing. Even modest gains in women's educational levels are associated with reduced fertility and lengthened intervals between pregnancies, resulting in improved measures of health (Caldwell, 1986). Education seems to provide a resource for giving women better control over their lives as well as the knowledge to care for their families and themselves. Improved opportunities for education, particularly for women, may prove to be the single most important tool for advancing health status in developing countries and elsewhere.

War and armed conflict are also determinants of health and of great public health concern. Under contemporary methods of engagement, it is increasingly the civilian population rather than the combatants themselves that account for the burden of direct casualties. Beyond the impacts of killing and direct injury are the consequences of disrupted economies, displacement of populations, inability to provide for basic human needs of food and shelter, and loss of basic sanitation. It is not surprising that war is associated with famine and epidemics. Public health agencies along with relief agencies have had to respond to enormous challenges spawned by wars and their aftermath. Unfortunately, public health has had little to offer in addressing the underlying causes of conflict such as rivalry, exaggerated nationalism, despotism, greed, and social and economic disparity. Even in the absence of active conflict, the buildup of arms diverts public resources needed for basic services.[1]

As noted previously (Chapter 4), the determinants and ecology of disease can be complex and are often incompletely perceived. Linkages among determinants often defy prediction and are recognized only in retrospect. For example, a transcontinental highway in Africa in combination with culturally prevalent patterns of male domination of sexual practices set the stage for rapid dissemination of HIV and contributed to the devastating epidemic of AIDS that would later engulf all major populations around the world. In contrast, the determinants of some diseases are well recognized. These diseases spread within the populations and across borders with predictability. Examples are the spread of enteric, respiratory, and other infections in association with crowding, poor sanitation, and poverty; the emergence of cardiovascular heart disease in association with development of national economies and adoption of diets high in animal fats, and sedentary lifestyles; and infections, malnutrition, and violence that occur with the generation of refugees in the face of war or oppression. The emergence of vaccine-preventable disease is a predictable consequence of disruption in public health infrastructure that can follow political destabilization, economic depression, and migration within the population. Figure 11.1 shows the effect on incidence of diphtheria following the dissolution of the Soviet Union.

Interactions between host, agent, and the environment extend beyond what is understandable through a biological model of disease. For example, the initial declines in rates of some of the historically important infections (e.g., tuberculosis) in industrialized countries preceded the institution of specific medical treatments (McKeown,

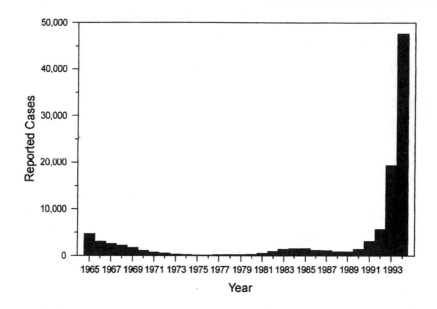

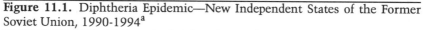

Figure 11.1. Diphtheria Epidemic—New Independent States of the Former Soviet Union, 1990-1994[a]
SOURCE: World Health Organization data; Centers for Disease Control and Prevention (1995c).
NOTE: a. Data for 1994 are provisional.

1979). The factors accounting for this phenomenon remain speculative, presumably involving improved housing and emergence of improved standards of living associated with economic growth.

The bases for the emergence of some new infections remain elusive. Researchers have been unable to explain the presumed adaptation of HIV from animal hosts to humans. The reasons for the episodic emergence of the Ebola virus in African locales are unknown.

Some problems emerge as a direct, unintended consequence of medical intervention. The inexorable emergence of antibiotic-resistant strains of virulent bacteria in settings where antibiotics are heavily used is an example. Specifically, the recent emergence of antibiotic-resistant strains of *M. tuberculosis* poses a major public health threat.

Demographic Transitions

Demographic transition refers specifically to the historical decline in fertility that has occurred in many developing countries. Demographic transition is associated with improvements in infant mortality and changes in age distribution in the population. Originally attributed to advances in maternal and infant health and to economic betterment, research has subsequently demonstrated that education of women has been the most important variable affecting fertility. This has an important implication for interventions in developing countries where lack of education perpetuates a cycle of high fertility, poverty, disease, infant mortality, and disempowerment.

Beyond reduction in fertility, there are other demographic changes that affect health. An example is global urbanization. In many resource-depleted rural areas, traditional subsistence lifestyles are no longer tenable and the associated poverty is no longer acceptable. Rapid urban migration is occurring in many countries. It is estimated that two thirds of the world's population will live in cities in the year 2015 (World Bank, 1993). Already, there are dozens of megacities having populations over 10 million.

Urbanization results in unfamiliar interdependence among people. Where economies are weak and infrastructure is underdeveloped, crowded living conditions, inadequate employment, and insufficient basic services, including lack of sanitation, transportation, and systems of communication, generate settings in which new and potentially massive health problems emerge.

On the other hand, stable economies and political structures have afforded many who live in urban areas access to education, food, housing, and other services. Unfortunately, the industrial production that drives the more developed economies also consumes resources, generates wastes, and often tolerates an impoverished underclass within its midst. Consequences include new exposures to occupational hazards, environmental toxins, and new social stresses.

Epidemiologic Transitions

In developing the concept of *epidemiologic transition,* Omran (1971) described a sequence of three distinct, historically identifiable stages: first, recurring cycles of epidemics and famine; then the receding of the pandemics; and ultimately, emergence of degenerative diseases and conditions related to environmental change. The transitions between each are characterized by profound changes in the incidence and patterns of disease and the causes of morbidity and mortality, and are tied directly to demographic transitions.

The declines in infectious disease and famine occur in the course of changing fertility and also changing standards of living, sanitation, access to food and immunization technologies, and methods to improve maternal and child health. The conspicuous transition from infectious to chronic disease is found in many developing countries, as well as in all developed countries—in particular, the emergence of cardiovascular disease, cancers, diabetes, and chronic lung disease. These conditions are associated with overnutrition, sedentary life styles, various environmental exposures, and tobacco use.

Epidemiologic transitions have occurred at different times and at different rates in various parts of the world. Changes in the incidence of chronic disease can occur with remarkable rapidity. This has been well documented among some indigenous populations, including Indian tribes in the southwestern United States. Within the span of just a few decades, there has been widespread emergence of obesity, high blood pressure, cardiovascular disease, and diabetes, with all the accompanying complications of these conditions.

Although the theory of epidemiologic transition as a sequence is complex, it provides a conceptual framework for viewing changes in patterns of disease and mortality. Specific instances of change may not exactly correspond with the theory. In some countries, concurrent with the emergence of chronic disease, children continue to have unacceptably high rates of malnutrition and infectious and parasitic disease. Inequalities in distributions of wealth and access to resources contribute to these situations. Although there have been improvements in infant and maternal mortality, child survival must continue as a priority for international assistance (Jamison & Mosley, 1991).

Another example of the complexity of transition is evident in contemporary contexts of urban migrations. Infectious diseases including tuberculosis, cholera, and AIDS, and nutritional problems coexist with the effects of alcohol and drug use, alienation and depression, domestic violence, assault, homicide, and suicide.

Globally, including developed countries where the risk of epidemic infection is perceived to be low, the threat or even the inevitability of new, emerging infectious diseases is real (Garrett, 1994). The emergence of HIV/AIDS provides a dramatic contemporary example. The emergence of the highly contagious, highly lethal, and untreatable Ebola virus infection in Africa is another example. The complex interplay among populations and their changing environments ensures a changing epidemiologic future that defies simple solution. It overwhelms, for example, any promise of overall health improvement that might be offered by access to medical services alone.

Priorities for International Health Assistance

The International Conference on Primary Health Care at Alma Ata in 1978 called for the attainment by all peoples of the world by the year 2000 of a level of health that will permit them to lead a socially and economically productive life. Improved access to primary health care was identified as the key in attaining this target (World Health Organization & United Nations Children's Fund, 1978). With the approach of the year 2000, it is now apparent that even this challenge for provision of basic health services will be out of reach for large portions of the world's population.

Taking a more sober assessment of health needs and their implications for policy, the *World Bank*, in its *Agenda for Action* has issued a broad guideline for investment in global health (World Bank, 1993, chap. 7). Categorizing needs separately for low- and middle-income nations, the World Bank has set forth varied agendas for each. For low-income countries, priority should be investment in infrastructure including education, public health services for the poor, reallocation of clinical services from tertiary to primary and preventive care, and increased community control of financing of services. Middle-income countries should focus on ensuring that public subsidies for health address needs of the poor rather than the better-off groups, and reforming insurance coverage to broaden coverage and promote efficiency. Needs and priorities rather than time lines are emphasized.

Emerging in the challenge offered with the declaration at Alma Ata and in the more recent *Agenda for Action* of the World Bank is the importance of developing basic infrastructure. Stable economies, an educated populace (particularly women), social justice in the distribution of services, efficiency of government, and local control in the allocation of financing for services are among the elements specifically cited.

A contrasting approach to developing infrastructure is to prioritize and target specific health problems. Categorical programs to control or eradicate individual diseases, correct nutritional deficiencies, provide access to family planning, and improve pregnancy outcomes are examples. The contrasting approaches are complementary. The categorical programs have succeeded in some arenas. The eradication of smallpox in the 1970s, the elimination of polio now from several continents, major advances in the control of measles and tuberculosis in many countries, and the curbing of rates of unwanted pregnancy in some countries have all been achieved through targeted programs using basic principles of public health.[2] These include sound epidemiologic analysis, scientifically based understanding of disease biology, rigorous surveillance and monitoring of health-related events, international cooperation and policy development, education and communication, and direct services. It is apparent, however, that targeted efforts are at high risk for failure without basic infrastructure and social stability. Community involvement is also essential for local participation with respect to implementation strategies.

Organization of International Assistance

Addressing health problems where they exist is a daunting task for public health. Limited willingness to allocate resources across international borders is one major reason. International initiatives that link assistance to political considerations can be detrimental.[3] Nevertheless, some U.S. governmental agencies such as the Centers for Disease Control and Prevention have provided valuable assistance, bringing technical resources to crises and situations of evolving emergency. Congress's mandate for the U.S. Agency for International Development (*USAID*) includes support for development of health services in underdeveloped countries. Analogous agencies exist in other countries.

The WHO, based in Geneva, and its affiliates, are constituted to provide neutral forums and means for global health assessment, prioritization, and program implementation. Constraints involve limited resources and the need to accommodate political sensitivities. WHO can do little without the full cooperation of the countries involved, which may not always be forthcoming. The United Nations Children's Fund (*UNICEF*) is mandated to address the particular needs of children. Another affiliated body is the United Nations High Commission on Refugees.

In addition, numerous nongovernmental organizations (*NGOs*) and religiously affiliated groups target aspects of the international and global health agenda. Individual NGOs are usually selective in the issues each will take on. Their contributions can be invaluable. The International Red Cross has a long history of providing rapid relief in settings of disaster. The Carter Center in Atlanta has been instrumental in the campaign to eradicate river blindness, a highly prevalent disease in parts of Africa and South America due to infection with the Guinea worm. NGOs can operate with relative independence from the global politics that constrain organizations such as WHO.

There are inherent tensions between community needs, national priorities, and donor assistance. Joining these in coordinated, mutually appreciated efforts to eradicate disease or improve health status continues to be a challenge.

Notes

1. At least one health organization has had an impact on the threat of war. The International Physicians for the Prevention of Nuclear War received the Nobel

Peace Prize in 1985 for its contributions in moving world powers toward nuclear disarmament. The U.S. affiliate organization is Physicians for Social Responsibility, which took a leadership role in this effort. (See Levy & Sidel, 1996, for more information in this area.)

2. Although there have been striking successes with some disease control programs, there have also been notable failures. One was the failed attempt to eradicate malaria. Tuberculosis has been controlled in some areas, but has spread in others. The emergence and spread of antibiotic-resistant tuberculosis in urban subpopulations in the United States is an example.

3. Agreements between the United States and some Asian countries with developing economies have been tied to allowance of the importation and marketing of American tobacco products in these countries. Although this helps U.S. trade balances and addresses regional economic issues within the United States, it undoubtedly is contributory to recent, marked increases in cigarette use and catastrophic increases projected for mortality from cardiovascular disease, as well as cancer and respiratory disease over the next three decades (Tominaga, 1986). In China alone, there may be 2 million tobacco-related deaths in 2025 as a result of the rapid increase in smoking during the 1980s (Peto, 1987).

Glossary of Terms

Absolute risk

The probability of a disease or condition occurring in a population.

Adjusted rate

The rate of occurrence of a disease or event, gathered from measures in a population that have been recomputed using a standard profile (e.g., age distribution).

Agent

That which specifically causes a disease or condition. For an infectious disease, it is the microbe. In environmental health, it is the toxin.

Assessment

One of the three core functions of public health practice; includes surveillance and monitoring, case-finding, needs analysis, forecasting trends, and evaluation of outcomes of interventions.

Assurance

One of the three core functions of public health practice; refers to providing services necessary to reach public health goals, either by encouraging (or requiring) private sector action or by providing services directly.

Attributable risk

That part of the total risk or incidence of a disease or condition that is due to a specific exposure or determinant.

Bias

In research, anything that introduces distortions such that results or conclusions will deviate systematically from the truth.

Blinded study

A research method in which either the subjects or the investigators (or both in a double blinded study) are unaware of which subjects are receiving or not receiving an intervention; used to reduce observation bias.

Block grant

A federal grant to a state or local agency to manage a specified program. The grantee usually has broad discretion in use of the funds.

Carcinogen

Any agent, especially a chemical, that causes cancer.

Cardiovascular disease (CVD)

A general category within which coronary heart disease is a sub-category.

Case

A person with a disease.

Case-control study

An epidemiologic study that seeks to determine the rate of prior exposure to a hypothesized causal determinant in persons known to have disease and compares this rate with the rate of exposure in persons without the disease. An odds ratio, which approximates relative risk, can be computed from such studies.

Case definition

A specific, operational definition used by epidemiologists to assign cases to a given diagnostic group.

Case report

Published description of a single clinical case, often used to suggest a hypothesis.

Categorical grant

More restrictive than a block grant, targeted at a specific disease, and with little local control.

Categorical program

A program organized and targeted on a specific disease or problem, for example, cancer or diabetes.

Cause

Anything that results in or contributes in an important way to the occurrence of an outcome. The causality of an association cannot be conclusively proven, but can be inferred when there is a coherent body of evidence that shows the association is strong and consistent, there is a gradient of effect corresponding to amount of exposure, temporality (the cause must precede the effect), plausibility, and experimental reproducibility.

Centers for Disease Control and Prevention (CDC)

An operating division of the Public Health Service within the Department of Health and Human Services; based in Atlanta, it supports health departments and conducts research and interventions with respect to diseases of public health importance.

Clinical trial

See controlled intervention.

Cohort

A study population that is followed over time.

Confidence interval

The statistically computed range around the average observed in the sample within which the true average of the population lies.

Confounding

When the true effect of one variable on an outcome is observed as distorted by the presence of a second (confounding) variable on the same outcome.

Control

A comparison group that reflects a baseline situation, for example, without the exposure in a cohort study, without the intervention in a controlled intervention, or without disease in a case-control study.

Controlled intervention

An experiment in which a study group receiving an intervention is followed prospectively to observe the effect of the intervention; results are compared with outcome in a control group.

Cross-sectional study

A study of a population in which information about the variables of interest is gathered at one point in time, often by a survey.

Crude rate

The rate of occurrence, determined directly from counts in the population.

Demographic transition

The decline in fertility that has occurred in developing countries, associated with improved infant mortality and changes in the distribution of population by age.

Department of Health and Human Services

A department of the federal government with multiple agencies and administrations that oversee regulation, operations, and financing of many federal health programs.

Determinant

An antecedent that contributes to change in health status.

Ecological study

Observations that correlate rates of occurrence of disease or events within populations with rates of occurrence of possibly associated variables within the same populations.

Effectiveness

The effect that an intervention actually achieves when applied in the real world, where circumstances preclude full efficacy.

Efficacy

The effect that an intervention can achieve when circumstances are optimally controlled to ensure full effect.

Environment

All domains outside of the person or population that can influence the person's or population's health. Domains include the physical, social, economic, and political environments.

Environmental Protection Agency (EPA)

An agency of the federal government with authority to regulate introduction of pollutants into the environment.

Epidemiologic transition

The historical sequence of change from epidemic diseases and famine to degenerative and chronic diseases caused by human activity that has occurred in association with the demographic transition.

Epidemiology

The study of distribution and determinants specific of health-related states or events in specified populations (Last, 1995, p. 55).

False positives

To the extent that a test is nonspecific, some of the instances of identified cases will in fact not be true cases. These are called false positives.

Food and Drug Administration (FDA)

An operating unit of the Public Health Service, having responsibility that includes approving drugs and safety of food additives and cosmetics in the United States.

Health

(a) A state of complete physical, mental, and social well-being, and not merely the absence of disease or infirmity (World Health Organization & United Nations Children's Fund, 1978). (b) The extent to which an individual or a group is able to realize aspirations and satisfy needs, and to change or cope with the environment. Health is a resource for everyday life, not the objective of living; it is a positive concept, emphasizing social and personal resources as well as physical capabilities (WHO, 1986, p. 426). (c) A state characterized by anatomic, physiologic and psychologic integrity; ability to perform personally valued family, work, and community roles; ability to deal with physical, biologic, psychologic, and social stress; a feeling of well-being; and freedom from the risk of disease and untimely death (Stokes, Noren, & Shindell, 1982).

Health Care Financing Administration (HCFA)

The federal agency within the Department of Health and Human Services responsible for administering Medicare and Medicaid and for certifying clinical laboratories.

Health maintenance organization (HMO)

A type of managed care organization that accepts prepayment to finance health services for enrollees.

Health promotion

(a) The process of enabling persons to increase control over, and to improve, their health (WHO, 1986). (b) Any planned combination of educational, political, regulatory, and organizational supports for actions and conditions of living conducive to the health of individuals, groups, or communities (Green & Kreuter, 1991, p. 432).

Health protection

Strategies of prevention that are external to the individual, created to shield (protect) the individual from harm, exposures, or other risks. Health protection is often implemented through laws and regulation.

Health Resources and Services Administration (HRSA)

An operating division of the Public Health Service in the Department of Health and Human Services.

Host

(a) Person in whom an infectious agent lodges and either persists and manifests itself as disease. (b) Person who is susceptible to having or actually has disease.

Human immunodeficiency virus (HIV)

The agent that causes AIDS.

Hypothesis

An tentative statement put forth to explain an observation or event, made to be tested through subsequent research.

Indian Health Service

An operating division of the Public Health Service in the Department of Health and Human Services.

Illness

The individual's experience or subjective perception of lack of physical or mental well-being, or both (Shah, 1994, p. 4).

Incidence

Rate of occurrence of new cases of a specified condition in a specified population within some time interval, usually a year.

Institute of Medicine (IOM)

A component of the National Academy of Sciences; published *The Future of Public Health*.

Managed care

The organization and delivery of health care services through organized systems that receive advanced payment (capitation) for each enrollee and assume the financial risk of covering the costs of care. Managed care organizations attempt to maintain quality of care and to control costs, including by limiting access to specialty services.

Managed care organization

A general term for any health plan delivering managed care services.

Medicaid

A federally mandated program, managed by individual states, to finance medical and behavioral, long-term care, and other health services for eligible, low-income people.

Medicare

A federally mandated program, financed through a special trust fund, principally to provide medical services for the elderly; also pays for renal dialysis.

Monitoring

The routine measurement of the status of occurrence of a disease to detect changes in the environment or in effectiveness of prevention and control programs.

Morbidity rate

A measure of the prevalence of disease or illness in living persons. It reflects the burden of suffering and disability, as opposed to death.

Mortality rate

A measure of the incidence of deaths in a population.

National Center for Health Statistics

A center within the CDC; conducts national surveys and assembles and publishes vital statistics and other health data.

National Health Service Corps

An agency administered by HRSA that places health professionals in medically underserved sites.

National Institutes of Health (NIH)

An operating division of the Public Health Service in the Department of Health and Human Services; conducts biomedical research.

Occupational Safety and Health Administration (OSHA)

An agency within the Department of Labor responsible for setting and enforcing standards for work site safety.

Pathogenesis

The causal process leading to a disease.

Placebo

A treatment or intervention having no biological effect; often given to control groups used to provide a reference for comparison in measuring the effectiveness of an intervention.

Policy

Statements that guide or regulate the activities of public or private agencies or organizations. Policy development is one of the three core functions of public health practice.

Population

(a) The inhabitants of a geographic unit. (b) Any specific group of people, defined in place and time and by characteristics, identified for purposes of analysis or planning.

Population attributable risk (PAR)

PAR is computed by multiplying the attributable risk by the prevalence in the population of those who are exposed, and dividing by the overall incidence.

Prevalence

The proportion of a specified population having a specified condition at a given point in time.

Prevention

Any strategy or activity designed to prevent disease or adverse health condition. Primary prevention is action taken to reduce incidence or risk of occurrence of disease. Secondary prevention is the screening and detection of disease in an early, presymptomatic stage to intervene, when prognosis is favorable. Tertiary prevention is intervention after disease has become manifest to reduce risk of recurrence or of complication.

Primary care

(a) Essential health care based on practical, scientifically sound and socially acceptable methods and technology made universally accessible to individuals and families in the community through their full participation and at a cost that the community and country can afford (World Health Organization & United Nations Children's Fund, 1978). (b) Medical care services for individuals that provide for management of many common conditions and preventive services, continuity of care, and referral to specialty care and hospitalization when needed.

Prognosis

Expected outcome of a disease (or condition or situation).

Prospective cohort study

A study design in which subjects (cohort) who have been exposed to a possible determinant or causal factor for disease are followed (prospectively) over time to determine outcome. Results are compared with outcome in a control group. Incidence and relative risk can be computed directly from the results.

Public health

A public enterprise having a mission to fulfill society's interest in ensuring the conditions in which people can be healthy, a structure comprised of organized community efforts aimed at the prevention of disease and promotion of health, and activities organized within both the formal structure of government and the associated efforts of private and voluntary organizations and individuals (Institute of Medicine, 1988, pp. 40-42).

Public Health Service

A part of the Department of Health and Human Services comprised of the Office of Public Health and Science, including its component offices, the Regional Health Administrators, and the following operating divisions: CDC, ATSDR, FDA, NIH, HRSA, IHS, Substance Abuse and Mental Health Services Administration-(SAMHSA), and Agency for Health Care Policy and Research (AHCPR).

p value

The measure of probability that an observed difference occurred by chance.

Quarantine

The isolation of a person during a period of possible infectivity to prevent spread of infectious disease, originally a period of 40 days.

Randomization

In research, a method of sampling or allocating in which each person in the population being studied has an equal chance of being included in the sample or allocation. Randomization is used to avoid selection bias and to ensure balanced distribution of characteristics across study groups.

Relative risk

A measure of the changed risk for a disease or condition as a result of some exposure, specifically the ratio of risk or incidence in the exposed group to the risk or incidence in an unexposed group.

Retrospective study

A study design in which the exposure to hypothesized antecedent determinants of disease is identified after the subjects with disease and their controls have been identified, as in a case-control study.

Risk

The probability that something will occur over the course of some period of time.

Risk factor

Anything that is directly or indirectly related to increased risk.

Sensitivity

A measure of the capability of a test finding all cases of a designated condition. It is computed as the number of true cases identified by the test divided by the total number of true cases in the tested population.

Sentinel condition

A designated disease or event, ordinarily preventable and of infrequent incidence, which is monitored because its occurrence may indicate a change in environment or other situation in which risk has increased and preventive intervention is needed.

Specificity

A measure of the capability of a test to identify noncases correctly. It is computed as the number of true negatives found by the test divided by the total number of noncases in the tested population.

Statistically significant

A measured difference may be statistically significant if the likelihood of its being due to chance (p value) is very low.

Statistics

Analytic tools that are essential for the applications of epidemiology and in the interpretation of data.

Surgeon general

Director of the Commissioned Corps of the U.S. Public Health Service; has assigned roles in setting directions and policies for the PHS.

Surveillance

The continuous search for the occurrence of a disease or condition to achieve early detection of outbreaks.

Syndrome

A group of symptoms or signs that constitute a specific diagnostic entity.

Vector

That which carries an agent to a host; important in disease transmission.

Vital records

Records compiled from birth and death certificates that permit tracking of population, natality statistics including birth complications, and mortality including causes of death.

Women, Infants, and Children Program (WIC)

A grants-in-aid program of the U.S. Department of Agriculture to states for supplemental nutrition and education for low-income pregnant women, postpartum mothers, and their young children.

World Bank

An organization comprised of member nations that finances loans to promote economic infrastructure and growth in developing countries.

World Health Organization (WHO)

An agency of the United Nations, based in Geneva, responsible for monitoring health in the countries of the world and initiating responses.

List of Acronyms

AIDS

Acquired immune deficiency syndrome

ATSDR

Agency for Toxic Substances and Disease Registry

CDC

Centers for Disease Control and Prevention

CHD

Coronary heart disease

CVD

Cardiovascular disease

DHHS

Department of Health and Human Services

EPA

Environmental Protection Agency

FDA

Food and Drug Administration

HCFA

Health Care Financing Administration

HIV

Human immunodeficiency virus

HMO

Health maintenance organization

HRSA

Health Resources and Services Administration

IHS

Indian Health Service

IOM

Institute of Medicine

MCO

Managed care organization

NGO

Nongovernmental organization

NIH

National Institutes of Health

NRC

Nuclear Regulatory Commission

OSHA

Occupational Safety and Health Administration

PAR

Population attributable risk

PHS

Public Health Service

UNICEF

United Nations Children's Fund

USAID

United States Agency for International Development

WHO

World Health Organization

WIC

Women, Infants, and Children Program

References

Ajzen, I. (1988). *Attitudes, personality, and behavior.* Chicago: Dorsey.

American Public Health Association. (1991). *Healthy communities 2000: Model standards, guidelines for community attainment of the year 2000 national health objectives.* Washington, DC: Author.

Angell, M. (1996). Evaluating the health risks of breast implants: The interplay of medical science, the law, and public opinion. *New England Journal of Medicine, 334,* 1513-1518.

Bandura, A. (1986). *Social foundations of thought and action: A social cognitive theory.* Englewood Cliffs, NJ: Prentice Hall.

Bennett, M. K. (1954). *The world's food.* New York: Harper.

Berkman, L. (1986). Social networks, support, and health: Taking the next step forward. *American Journal of Epidemiology, 123,* 559-561.

Bettman, J. R. (1979). *Information processing theory of consumer choice.* Reading, MA: Addison-Wesley.

Caldwell, J. C. (1986). Routes to low mortality in poor countries. *Population and Development Review, 12,* 171-220.

Canadian Task Force on the Periodic Health Examination. (1979). The periodic health examination. *Canadian Medical Association Journal, 121*(9), 1193-1254.

Centers for Disease Control and Prevention. (1986). *Comprehensive plan for epidemiologic surveillance.* Atlanta, GA: Author.

Centers for Disease Control and Prevention. (1993). Outbreak of acute illness—Southwestern United States. *Morbidity and Mortality Weekly Report, 42,* 421-424.

Centers for Disease Control and Prevention. (1995a). *Fact book, 1995.* Atlanta, GA: Author.

Centers for Disease Control and Prevention. (1995b). *Planned approach to community health: Guide for the local coordinator.* Atlanta, GA: U.S. Department of Health and Human Services, Public Health Service.

Centers for Disease Control and Prevention. (1995c). Diphtheria epidemic—New independent states of the former Soviet Union, 1990-1994. *Morbidity and Mortality Weekly Report, 44,* 177-181.

Centers for Disease Control and Prevention. (1996a). Births and deaths: United States, 1995. *Monthly Vital Statistics Report, 45*(3, Suppl. 2).

Centers for Disease Control and Prevention. (1996b). Addition of prevalence of cigarette smoking as a nationally notifiable disease. *Morbidity and Mortality Weekly Report, 45,* 537.

Centers for Disease Control and Prevention. (1996c). Surveillance for Creutzfeldt-Jakob disease—United States. *Morbidity and Mortality Weekly Report, 45*(31), 665-668.

Centers for Disease Control and Prevention. (1996d). Changes in national notifiable diseases data presentation. *Morbidity and Mortality Weekly Report, 45*(2), 41-42.

Centers for Disease Control and Prevention. (1996e). Progress toward elimination of *Haemophilus influenzae* type b disease among infants and children. *Morbidity and Mortality Weekly Report, 45*(42), 901-906.

Centers for Disease Control and Prevention. (1997a). Estimated expenditures for core public health functions. *Morbidity and Mortality Weekly Report, 46*(7), 150-152.

Centers for Disease Control and Prevention. (1997b). Angiosarcoma of the liver among polyvinyl chloride workers. *Morbidity and Mortality Weekly Report, 46*(5), 97-101.

Duhl, L. J. (1993). Conditions for healthy cities; diversity, game board, and social entrepreneurs. *Environment and Urbanization, 5*(2), 112-124.

Epp, J. (1986). *Achieving health for all: A framework for health promotion.* Ottawa, Canada: Report of the Minister of National Health and Welfare.

Evans, R. G., Barer, M. L., & Marmor, T. R. (Eds.). (1994). *Why are some people healthy and others not? The determinants of health of populations.* Hawthorn, NY: Aldine de Gruyter.

Fishbein, M., & Ajzen, I. (1975). *Belief, attitude, intention, and behavior: An introduction to theory and research.* Reading, MA: Addison-Wesley.

Freire, P. (1970). *Pedagogy of the oppressed.* New York: Seabury.

Garrett, L. (1994). *The coming plague: Newly emerging diseases in a world out of balance.* New York: Penguin.

Gilmore, G., & Campbell, M. D. (1996). *Needs assessment strategies for health education and health promotion.* Madison, WI: Brown & Benchmark.

Green, L. W., & Kreuter, M. W. (1991). *Health promotion planning: An educational and environmental approach* (2nd ed.). Mountain View, CA: Mayfield.

Health Care Financing Administration. (1997). *Office of the Actuary: Data from the Office of National Health Statistics.* (Available from HCFA, telephone: [410] 786-6374)

Hecker, J. (1839). *The epidemics of the Middle Ages.* London: Trubner.

Hertzman, P. A., Blevins, W. L., Mayer, J., Greenfield, B., Ting, M., & Gleich, G. J. (1990). Association of eosinophilia-myalgia syndrome with ingestion of tryptophan. *New England Journal of Medicine, 322,* 869-873.

Hill, A. B. (1965). *Principles of medical statistics* (9th ed.). New York: Oxford University Press.

Hunink, M. G. M., Goldman, L., Tosteson, A. N. A., Mittleman, M. A., Goldman, P. A., Williams, L. W., Tsevat, J., & Weinstein, M. C. (1997). The recent decline in mortality from coronary heart diseases. *Journal of the American Medical Association, 277*(7), 535-542.

Institute of Medicine. (1988). *The future of public health.* Washington, DC: National Academy Press.

Institute of Medicine. (1996). *Healthy communities: New partnerships for the future of public health.* Washington, DC: National Academy Press.

Jamison, D. T., & Mosley, W. H. (1991). Disease control priorities in developing countries: Health policy responses to epidemiological change. *American Journal of Public Health, 81*(1), 15-22.

Joint Committee on Health Education Terminology. (1991). Report of the 1990 joint committee on health education terminology. *Journal of Health Education, 22*(2), 97-108.

Labonte, R. (1993). *Issues in health promotion series. Number 3: Health promotion and empowerment. Practice frameworks.* Toronto, Canada: University of Toronto, Centre for Health Promotion.

Lalonde, M. (1974). *A new perspective on the health of Canadians.* Ottawa: Government of Canada.

Last, J. M. (1987). *Public health and human ecology.* East Norwalk, CT: Appleton-Lange.

Last, J. M. (1992). Ethics and public health policy. In J. M. Last & R. B. Wallace (Eds.), *Maxcy Rosenau–Last public health preventive medicine* (13th ed., pp. 1187-1196). Norwalk, CN: Appleton-Lange.

Last, J. M. (Ed.). (1995). *A dictionary of epidemiology* (3rd ed.). New York: Oxford.

Lefebvre, C., & Flora, J. (1988). Social marketing and public health intervention. *Health Education Quarterly, 15,* 299-315.

Levy, B. S., & Sidel, V. W. (Eds.). (1996). *War and public health.* New York: Oxford University Press.

MacMahon, B., & Trichopoulos, D. (1996). *Epidemiology principles and methods* (2nd ed.). Boston: Little, Brown.

Marmot, M. G., Kogevinas, M., & Elston, M. A. (1987). Social/economic status and disease. *Annual Review of Public Health, 8,* 111-135.

McGinnis, J. M., & Foege, W. H. (1993). Actual causes of death in the United States. *Journal of the American Medical Association, 270*(18), 2207-2212.

McKeown, T. (1979). *The role of medicine: Dream, mirage, or nemesis?* (2nd ed.). Oxford, UK: Basil Blackwell.

McNeill, W. (1989). *Plagues and people.* New York: Doubleday.

Mercy, J. A., Rosenberg, M. L., Powell, K. E., Broome, C. V., & Roper, W. L. (1993, Winter). Public health policy for preventing violence. *Health Affairs, 12,* 7-29.

Merriam Webster's collegiate dictionary (9th ed.). (1990). Springfield, MA: Merriam-Webster.

Minkler, M. (1995). Building supportive ties and sense of community among inner-city elderly: The Tenderloin Senior Outreach project. *Health Education Quarterly, 12*(4), 303-314.

Murray, C. J. L., & Lopez, A. D. (1996). Evidence-based health policy—Lessons from the global burden of disease study. *Science, 274,* 740-743.

National Cancer Institute. (1995). *Theory at a glance: A guide for health promotion practice* (NIH Publication No. 95-3996). Bethesda, MD: National Institutes of Health.

Omran, A. R. (1971). The epidemiologic transition: A theory of the epidemiology of population change. *Milbank Memorial Fund Quarterly, 49,* 509-538.

Palmer, R., & Colton, J. (1995). *A history of the modern world* (8th ed.). New York: Knopf.

Pearce, N. (1996). Traditional epidemiology, modern epidemiology, and public health. *American Journal of Public Health, 86,* 678-683.

Peto, R. (1987). Tobacco-related deaths in China [Letter]. *Lancet, 2*(8552), 211.

Preston, J. (1996, April 14). Hospitals look on charity care as unaffordable option of past. *The New York Times, National Edition,* pp. A1, A15.

Reynolds, H. (n.d.). *Alar and a case of misinformation* [On-line]. Available: http://sib.lrs.uoguelph.ca/d1\alar.htm

Richardson, B. (1887). *The health of nations, a review of the works of Edwin Chadwick.* London: Longmans, Green.

Roemer, M. I. (1985). *National strategies for health care organization.* Ann Arbor, MI: Health Administration Press.

Rosen, G. (1993). *A history of public health* (expanded ed.). Baltimore, MD: Johns Hopkins University.

Rosenstock, I. M., Strecher, V. J., & Becker, M. (1988). Social learning theory and the health belief model. *Health Education Quarterly, 15*(2), 175-183.

Rothman, J., & Tropman, J. E. (1987). Models of community organization and macro practice: Their mixing and phasing. In F. M. Cox, J. L. Ehrlich, J. Rothman, & J. E. Tropman (Eds.), *Strategies for community organization: Macro practice* (4th ed., pp. 3-26). Itasca, IL: Peacock.

Ruckelshaus, W. D. (1983). Science risk and public policy. *Science, 221,* 1025-1028.

Rush, D., Horvitz, D., Seaver, W., Alvir, J., Garbowski, G., Leighton, J., Sloan, N., Johnson, S., Kulka, R., & Shankin, D. (1988). The national WIC evaluation: Evaluation of the Special Supplemental Food Program for women, infants, and children. *American Journal of Clinical Nutrition, 48*(Suppl. 2), 389-393.

Russell, L. (1986). *Is prevention better than cure?* Washington, DC: Brookings Institute.

Russell, L. (1986). *Is prevention better than cure?* Washington, DC: Brookings Institute.

Rutstein, D. D., Berenberg, W., Chalmers, T. C., Child, C. G., III, Fisherman, A. P., & Perrin, E. B. (1976). Measuring the quality of medical care; a clinical method. *New England Journal of Medicine, 294,* 582-588.

Selikoff, I. J., & Hammond, E. C. (1979). Asbestos and smoking [Editorial]. *Journal of the American Medical Association, 242,* 458-459.

Shah, C. P. (1994). *Public health and preventive medicine in Canada* (3rd ed.). Toronto, Canada: University of Toronto.

Slovic, P. (1987). Perception of risk. *Science, 236*(4799), 280-285.

Stokes, J., III, Noren J. J., & Shindell, S. (1982). Definition of terms and concepts applicable to clinical preventive medicine. *Journal of Community Health, 8*(1), 33-41.

Susser, M., & Susser, E. (1996). Choosing a future for epidemiology: II. From black box to Chinese boxes and eco-epidemiology. *American Journal of Public Health, 86,* 674-677.

Tabbush, V., & Swanson, G. (1996, February 26). Changing paradigms in medical payment. *Archives of Internal Medicine, 156*(4), 357-360.

Tengs, T. O., Adams, M. E., Pliskin, J. S., Safran, D. G., Siefel, J. E., Weinstein, M. C., & Graham, J. D. (1995). Five hundred life-saving interventions and their cost-effectiveness. *Risk Analysis, 15*(3), 369-390.

Terris, M. (1985). The public health profession. *Journal of Public Health Policy, 6*(1), 7-14.

Testa, M. A., & Simonson, D. C. (1996). Assessment of quality-of-life outcomes. *New England Journal of Medicine, 334*(13), 835-840.

Tominaga, S. (1986). Spread of smoking to the developing countries. In D. G. Zaridze & R. Peto (Eds.), *Tobacco: A major international health hazard* (International Agency for Research on Cancer Scientific Publication No. 74, pp. 125-133). New York: Oxford.

Tsouros, A. D. (1995). The WHO Healthy Cities project: State of the art and future plans. *Health Promotion International, 10*(2), 133-141.

U.S. Department of Health and Human Services. (1980). *Promoting health/preventing disease: Objectives for the nation.* Washington, DC: Public Health Service.

U.S. Department of Health and Human Services. (1989). *Reducing the health consequences of smoking: 25 years of progress, a report of the Surgeon General* (DHHS Publication No. CDC 89-8411). Washington, DC: Author.

U.S. Department of Health and Human Services. (1990). *Healthy people 2000: National health promotion and disease prevention objectives* (PHS Publication No. 91-50212). Washington, DC: Public Health Service.

U.S. Department of Health, Education, and Welfare. (1964). *Smoking and health* (Report of the Advisory Committee to the Surgeon General of the Public Health Service, PHS Publication No. 1103). Washington, DC: Public Health Service.

U.S. Department of Health, Education, and Welfare. (1979). *Healthy people: Surgeon general's report on health promotion and disease prevention* (PHS Publication No. 79-55071). Washington DC: Public Health Service.

U.S. Preventive Services Task Force. (1996). _Guide to clinical preventive services_ (2nd ed.). Baltimore, MD: Williams & Wilkins.

van Ryn, M., & Heaney, C. A. (1992). What's the use of theory? _Health Education Quarterly, 19_(3), 315-330.

Wallack, L., Dorfman, L., Jernigan, D., & Themba, M. (1993). Improving health prevention: Media advocacy and social marketing approaches. In L. Wallack, L. Dorfman, D. Jernigan, & M. Themba (Eds.), _Media advocacy and public health_ (pp. 1-25). Newbury Park, CA: Sage.

Wallerstein, N. (1992). Powerlessness, empowerment, and health: Implications for health promotion programs. _American Journal of Health Promotion, 6_(3), 197-205.

Ware, J. E., Jr., & Sherbourne, C. D. (1992). The MOS 36-item short-form health survey (SF-36). I. Conceptual framework and item selection. _Medical Care, 30,_ 473-483.

Wilkinson, R. G. (1992). Income distribution and life expectancy. _British Medical Journal, 304,_ 165-168.

Will, R. G., Ironside, J. W., Seidler, M., Cousens, S. N., Estibeiro, K., Alperovitch, A., Poser, S., Pocchiar, M., Hofman, A., & Smith, P. G. (1996). A new variant of Creutzfeldt-Jakob disease in the U.K. _Lancet, 347,_ 921-925.

Williams, R. (1951). _The United States Public Health Service 1798-1950._ Washington, DC: Commissioned Officers Association of the United States Public Health Service.

Winslow, C. (1920). The untilled field of public health. _Modern Medicine, 2,_ 183.

Witmer, A., Seifer, S., Finnocchio, L., Leslie, J., & O'Neil, E. (1995). Community health workers: Integral members of the health care workforce. _American Journal of Public Health, 85_(8), 1055-1058.

World Bank. (1993). _World development report 1993, Investing in health._ New York: Oxford University Press.

World Health Organization. (1944). The Constitution of the World Health Organization. _WHO Chronicle, 1,_ 29.

World Health Organization. (1983). _New approaches to health education in primary health care: Report of a WHO expert committee_ (WHO Tech. Rep. Series 690). Geneva: Author.

World Health Organization. (1984). _Health promotion: A discussion document._ Copenhagen, Denmark: Author.

World Health Organization. (1986). A charter for health promotion (Ottawa charter). _Canadian Journal of Public Health, 77,_ 425-430.

World Health Organization. (1995). _World health report 1995_ [On-line]. Available: http://www.who.ch/programmes/whr/whr_home.htm

World Health Organization and United Nations Children's Fund. (1978). _Primary health care: Report of international conferences at Alma Ata._ Geneva: World Health Organization.

Index

About the Authors

Jo Fairbanks, Ph.D., is currently teaching in the Masters in Public Health degree program at the University of New Mexico. In addition to extensive classroom experience, she has also spent many years in public health practice.

William H. Wiese, M.D., M.P.H., is Professor Emeritus, Department of Family and Community Medicine at the University of New Mexico School of Medicine. He is cofounder of the public health program at the University of New Mexico. He is presently Director of the Division of Public Health in the New Mexico Department of Health.